Self-Care

the real story of healing

Michelle Brenner

Copyright © 2022 Michelle Brenner

The information in this book is not to be seen as medical advice or seen to be a substitute to professional guidance. Neither the publisher nor the author take responsibility beyond the intention of this book as an inspiration and narrative of a real life experience and the existing literature that goes someway in explaining the what the why and how.

All rights reserved.

ISBN 979-8-78-910867-3

DEDICATION

To my children Golda and Joel

CONTENTS

Acknowledgement		Pg	9
Chapter	1	Pg	11
Chapter	2	Pg	25
Chapter	3	Pg	43
Chapter	4	Pg	65
Chapter	5	Pg	81
Chapter	6	Pg	101
About the author		Pg	115
Endnotes		Pg	117

ACKNOWLEDGEMENT

From the moment I realized I was not able to move my back, my core self, I saw a fork in the road. The slippery slope down or the mysterious journey up. My first thank you is for my son, Joel, for reminding me so quickly about the richness of self-care, initialy via the homeopathic stash that is in my study. That first choice took my breathing out of total shock to calm. Thank you to all the wonderful scientists, physicians, authors and journalists who have taken the time, research and effort to make self-care a real pathway. They are too many to list and they are really what this book is about. Honoring their life's work to enable us all to make healthy choices makes life so much more enjoyable.

Satchin Panda and Fred Luskin, at different times in my life, both responded to my emails and questions, again showing up in real life helping me to continue down this path of empowerment. Thank you to Reverend Somaloka, who, many years ago suggested I study natural therapies including homeopathy, and more recently showed me a paper he wrote some 20 years ago that introduced me to Dr Herbert Benson and Dr David Hamilton. The power of the placebo and nocebo are not just thinking is believing and believing is becoming, but also show the power of action. In the act of taking a pill, the body expects to be soothed, just like a baby will stop crying when it sees its mother, or is picked up. Magic happens when we have had safe experiences beforehand.

I am so grateful for all the teachers and workshops, training, and courses I have done over the last 35 years that have given me ways, tools and insight into well-being. It is with the gift of life and wellness that I have benefited from nature, the beaches that enable swimming to be easy, and the air to breathe. Bruce Stark has been my Ortho-Bionomy mentor and instructor, I knew that whatever condition I was going to be left in, I knew that Bruce would be there to help. Just knowing that made my choices so much easier.

Rod Lee is my Tai Chi teacher, and I am very grateful to him for bringing the practice of slow into my life. Rabbi Perlow, was critical as part of my support network. Thank you to Rabbi Eli Feldman who came to see me in hospital, the only visitor I could have in lockdown, he is a hospital chaplain. My daughter Golda, took over my life when I couldn't do what I usually do, and she stepped in and up beautifully. Miriam, and Sally Anne, organized so much behind the scenes and made me feel loved. Being loved mattered more than I can say. Love is really behind wellness and particularly behind self-care. It is not a taken for granted in life, and when it is there, I am so grateful to whoever brings it.

CHAPTER 1

Its Friday morning, September 17, 2021, Sydney. The date is significant because its during COVID 19 lockdown, a time we who live in Sydney Australia will always look back on as 'time inside'. I am looking out the window. The sun is bringing light to my eyes and I see the tops of bare trees, gently moving. A little bird, a bird with a deep round full chest is hopping from one branch to another. It looks playful, healthy and peaceful. Another bird, looking the same is hopping next to it, looks like it's wanting to be close but the first bird I noticed hops away each time the second bird comes near. I continue looking on, and eventually bird number two gives up. Bird number one is again at peace gently swaying with the branch under it as the wind blows.

I am lying in bed, on the seventh floor. The trees must be very tall, I see the tops and I never realized how high little birds fly and perch. I can't move my back, I had an accident at home, in the late afternoon the day before. I slipped down the last three steps of my inside stairwell. I am lying here after a night in the emergency and I am still traumatized, that is unable to move most of my body, just my feet and hands. I can't move my back, it doesn't follow my instinct that usually exists. I am not by the window, there are three other people in the room, and I feel like a newcomer. The window is the whole wall but curtains keep me from the greater part of the light. My instinct tells me to open the curtains, but I quickly realize I can't. Physically I cannot walk to the light, the window, I am dependent on asking others and when I see the others, nobody seems to care that a lot of light is hidden. I ask a nurse if she can open the curtain to increase the sunlight into the room and now, I am able to see more of the trees.

Compared to the way I feel, the bird and the tree look fully alive, and beautiful. They seem to mirror the energy that brings the sunlight to my eyes. I am reminded of the words of Mindfulness teacher Jon Kabat Zinn "if you can breathe, there is more right with you than wrong with you."[1] Yes, I can breathe, not move, but my breathing is great.

Even while I write this on my computer, weeks later, I can only sit for what seems like half a paragraph before the ache and discomfort in sitting gives way to me needing to lie down. The reason I want to tell this story of what happened at this time in my life, is because the story reveals so much strength, strength that is hidden in the world of pain and trauma.

Let's go back to my life before the slip, the slip actually wasn't the worst, the worst was the traumas that followed, the pain of movement, the news of a broken spine, the news of things wrong, pain to come and the realization that I have been traumatized and now am intolerant of and anticipating hurt and pain.

Trauma is defined by the American Psychological Association as

> "an emotional response to a terrible event like an accident, rape or natural disaster. Immediately after the event, shock and denial are typical. "

Shock, yes, I was and still am a few weeks later still feeling shock. The first instance of shock was noticing the sense of my back knocking against the edge of the stair and the unexplainable sense of my body shutting down. Luckily, I had my son next to me, and when he said, "Mum, are you okay?" I remember thinking, I don't know, I really don't know if I am okay."

One of the best parts of my life is being known, that I am not a stranger all the time. Although there is joy in freshness with novel experiences and discovering new people and places, there is a profound depth in appreciation which comes from a shared past, a knowing that has taken place where kindness was given and been received. An appreciation that comes from memories of being known. My son immediately asked if he should get the Arnica, a homeopathic remedy for falls and sprains. He grew up knowing that natural therapies are my first port of call for both mind and body symptoms. I was a homeopath, natural health therapist and conflict resolution consultant before he was born, I have for the last 35 years been continuously studying and practicing natural remedies for mind and body. Having worked with government at different levels, families, community groups and individuals.

Work included body function, relationship issues, hurts and losses; work place dramas with police and schools. At one point I moved from conflict to focusing on teaching, writing and working with positive energy, mostly my own. I remember ordering the book The Psychology of Gratitude a compilation of chapters by academics edited by Robert A. Emmons and Michael E. McCullough in 2004 when it first came out. This book revolutionised the age of wisdom that kindness was not just a moral attribute but a scientifically tested characteristic that impacts and enhances one's life at a body level not just a mind one.

At one stage in my career, I taught the subject Advanced Mediation at the University of Technology in Sydney (UTS) as part of the Masters in Alternative

Dispute Resolution. Work and personal development were interrelated as I would take home what I learnt as a mediator and community facilitator. Natural therapies for the body were put aside whilst my career path in mediation and community facilitation took precedent. I was always researching, looking for answers to questions that I would find in my work.

For instance, there was a time around 2007 when a couple came to me for mediation. They had been married eighteen years, had two beautiful boys, one eight years old and the other boy was six years old. The mother came from the Philippines and the father was a tall blonde Australian. After meeting with the couple twice, I realised that the bridge between them had become a gulf, almost like strangers they would sit, disinterested in what the other had to say.

When I spoke to the husband alone, I asked him if there was something that had happened that hadn't been brought up so far. He told me that on their wedding night, his wife told him that she had a son, that he was then five years old and that he lived in Darwin. He said to me, "How could I trust her from then? On our wedding night I find out that she had kept such a secret from me. Now how could I trust her." He continued. "What would you do if someone tricked you like that?"

This man had acute psoriasis, a skin inflammation that is triggered by stress. Eighteen years of knowing that his wife had born a son and not mentioned it until their wedding night became literally a thorn in his side. He was on pain killers that meant his thinking was affected. Pain killers are designed to be a barrier to pain, and part of the side effects of the barrier is reduced thinking. I could tell from our first meeting that we needed to go slow and be very clear with what was being said, and heard. It was evident from years of working with people in conflict that processing feeling and thoughts was not easy during stressful times, and alcohol, drugs including pain killers made processing even more difficult.

There are many ways in supporting people to process feelings and thoughts. Both one's own as well as others. One way I had discovered was storytelling. Lived experiences that came from research and personal life, support understanding and making sense of otherwise chaotic or rigid thinking. I took a moment and thought. Yes, I had come across infidelity, disloyalty, crossing a moral line and watched others navigate with this experience. What were the outcomes, the ways people had continued? I remembered hearts broken, trust damaged, pain felt and then started to think of the variety of futures these produced. I realised that some people separated and kept the pain and hurt inside them, while others stayed together and the hurt was buried under work, or other busy ness. Then other people I had come across let the pain dissolve, healing their hurt, moving away from holding onto the awful memory and when I remembered these people, some had separated and yet others stayed together. What was at the heart of healing injustice? It seemed to be forgiveness. A word not often used in law and dispute resolution, a word I connected rather to religion. With these thoughts, I said, "Could you forgive her?" his response, "How can I forgive her, could you, if this happened to you?"

Again, I was asked to consider the difficulty, how could and would a person forgive something that feels unforgivable? Not easily, I realised, not without guidance in 'how' to forgive. This took me on a research drive, which uncovered work by Fred Luskin director of the Stanford University Forgiveness Projects at Stanford University, California as well as to Hawaii where Forgiveness Day under the direction of Roger Epstein, was taken as a way of healing community hurts.

In short, the learnings that came from this became part of the next years Advanced Mediation subject at UTS, as well as the basis of the Assertive Communication course I taught at the City East Community College. This then became the first book I published Conscious Connectivity, Creating dignity in conversation.

Forgiveness is firstly about being curious about what is the hurt, the physical sensations that our body feels as well as the emotional hurt that comes as a result of injustice, whether the injustice is easy to see or not.

Sometimes we are sensing pain whilst at other times deny its presence or dismiss it. In many cases the injustice is hidden, located behind culture or normal practices. This can cause us to hide from our own pain, discount it as though it is not there. This then begins a sense of separating parts of ourselves from our full selves, our wholeness reshapes into separate parts, parts we embrace, and parts we disassociate from. Being curious and naming the hurt in our body as well as in hearts, is the first stage of forgiveness, being able to notice and name our pain is a critical stage in being well.

Well-being, Professor Felicia Huppert Professor of Psychology Emeritus, University of Cambridge; Honorary Professor, Body, Heart and Mind in Business Research Group at The University of Sydney says, is' having an open mind, an open heart and clear thinking.'[2] When part of us is closed or shut down from hurt or pain, we are not able to be truly open. Openness refers to being open to others as well as to ourselves. To be open is to have others see us as we are on the inside and for us to be curious of the inner worlds of others. The opposite of open is closed, off limits and blind to what is there. Noticing and identifying hurt and pain in our bodies and our feelings, is the first part of healing. Being able to let go requires a knowing of what and where it is that needs to be let go. By putting our attention on where is the pain, what is it that really disturbs us, there is a sort of light on, albeit a soft light. This enables clarity, what was hidden becomes seen and with wise compassion can be ushered into awareness. Sometimes we can do this ourselves but often we need others to support us.

Most of us go about our lives disconnected from parts of our bodies and parts of our emotions. Attending to our pain is not an easy task, sometimes the pain is too much to investigate, sometimes it feels so pervasive it doesn't have a place, it is everywhere. Often our attention is habitually outwardly directed and it feels foreign to check into ourselves.

Western culture and especially modern culture play a strong role in placing our attention outside of us. We are shaped in modern society to see that value comes from the manmade world, in the guise of technology and expertise in academia known via separate disciplines.

Prior to the industrial revolution people lived in communities that relied mostly on themselves. Whatever expertise existed within a geographical location was highly valued and regarded. Communities became known for the cultures that were held dear. If someone was interested in developing outside this understanding they travelled by foot, by horse or camel or by boat to other communities. Word of mouth became the marker for information. It would often be the word of mouth by an outsider or a returning soul that would bring news. Books were either non-existent or rare and word of mouth and foot travelling was how knowledge was shared. This required conversations, meetings and greetings between people that essentially was social engagement.

As the industrial revolution took hold and books, newspapers and universities, trains and technology developed, the human foot and mouth became less important. Expertise became more and more situated outside the human being. Expertise became so valued that it became profitable, commercial. Fast forward to the middle of the 20th century and expertise became only situated outside of humans or nature.

Whether it is that we go to a doctor to discover what is 'wrong' with our bodies, or get a professional trainer to 'guide' us to get fit, or a psychologist to council us in relationship issues. These practices are scientifically evaluated and assessed via expertise, often technological expertise that relates to professional qualifications. Modern Culture gained a reputation for being professionally and objectively scientifically driven. However, as I discovered, traditional cultures, indigenous societies, had a history of knowing that had continued through word of mouth by oral bearers that was full of working practices and social wisdom which lead to healing.

Natural therapies, which was my first career pursuit; was not taught in universities or science-based areas of study. They were more like crafts, apprenticeship style learnings that came from India, Hawaii, Japan, as well as Germany and other countries, I had initially discovered these whilst living in Hawaii, Japan and Indonesia, watching how local country people cared for each other and their own health. Expertise in less industrialised cultures, I noticed was connected to tradition, wisdom practices as well as adapting towards modern social norms.

When I moved into the field of Conflict Resolution, I became familiar with restorative justice but it wasn't till I returned to Hawaii in 2009 to be part of their Forgiveness Day that I discovered that restorative justice, also known as reintegrative justice was actually taken from indigenous people in Hawaii, New Zealand and native Canadian Indians, the 1st world nations. What I learnt from traditional oral bearers was holistic, it wasn't based on what was done but rather who one is. By being in tune with healing energy one becomes a conduit for healing to be present. So much of the practice is in preparation for tuning into positive healing energy.

At around this time, the early part of the 21st century, integrative research became popular in academia. More and more people from separate areas of research were interested in joining with other academic disciplines asking the same questions and looking at a variety of ways these questions could be seen rather than continuing down separate isolated pathways.

Integrative medicine became known more commonly as Complimentary Medicine, recognising that the modern world of medicine could be complimented by the traditional or alternative world of therapies that were not part of the registered medicine word view.

By the late 1990's a new discipline was being taught in universities all over the world. The theories and practice of Conflict Resolution acknowledged the interdisciplinary nature of knowledge. As Conflict Resolution situates itself in a practical arena, the curiosity of what worked in the past and what didn't, opens up space for inquisitiveness. I was very comfortable in recognising how the traditional wisdom of our ages can sit with modern expertise. Not always needing to be side by side, often it is one or the other at different times.

Getting back to lying on the floor in my house when my son asks me if am I alright, I wondered what the answer was. The Arnica had stopped my galloping heart rate and lack of being able to talk or think. I could not move though, that I could tell. I could wiggle my toes and my fingers but felt my back was stuck, motionless and unable to move. I positioned myself in a way that limited pain and thought. Okay, I can stay here till I feel better.

In the end the ambulance was called and the young lady paramedics who came insisted I go to Hospital. I remember saying, I am okay at home, I knew that

COVID 19 was still part of our community and we were still in lockdown. Hospital was not a place I wanted to be for a few reasons. I remember telling the paramedic, "I am fine on the floor, I have lived in Japan, everything we did was on the floor, I am very comfortable on the floor." It was Yom Kippur, the holiest day of the year, I had fasted all day, and did not need to go to the toilet. I thought a couple of days on the floor, not moving may be all that is needed to be okay. However, this wasn't seen as reasonable.

After discussion around leaving me on the floor or going to hospital we agreed the paramedics would lift me to the dining room chair. If I could sit there, I could stay at home. On the count of three, I was lifted and with a pain that I found unimaginable I was put on the chair. I was reexperiencing the agony, the excruciating sense that I was broken and the desire to be replaced on the floor flooded my body. Back on the floor it was understood, something was wrong and we needed the hospital to identify it. No, I could not move again onto a rolling chair that would take me outside to be transferred onto the ambulance stretcher, no way could I tolerate movement.

To get to the hospital I was given a 'green whistle'. A deep breath in and I left my body. I was in the sky, they could do what they wanted with my body, it was no longer part of my world. With this green whistle I was a spirit watching the clouds and tops of trees pass by, the colour of the sky changed and the stars appeared. I was pain free.

CHAPTER 2

Once in the hospital I was again awake to my situation. After being tested for COVID, (I had already had my vaccinations) and my blood pressure, temperature and oxygen levels taken I was placed very carefully on a trauma bed and wheeled for various tests. I vaguely remember these. I do recall repeating I did not want to moved. I could not move my body and was very afraid of anyone transferring me. I was given pain killer medication but I had no trust in anyone touching me. When I was told I was going to have a Magnetic Resonance Imaging scan, which is a medical imaging technique used in radiology to form pictures of the anatomy and the physiological processes of the body, I remember checking that I did not have to be moved, checking that I could remain on the trauma bed. But when I got to the scanner, they wanted to shift me. I asked the staff if they had another green whistle, but they were not nurses, they were radiographers. No, they had no medication, hence I refused to be shifted and was returned back to the emergency. Eventually a different person came to my side, who was wearing green, was kind and interested in me, I thought he was a doctor. When he said, he wanted to take me to get scanned, I trusted his soft approach and told him I could not be moved, the pain was too intense and his assurance around the way he would do it, softened my fear. So off I went, under his gentle guidance. It turned out he was not a doctor, rather a very kind hospital patient mover.

Eventually a doctor introduced himself as a neurosurgeon, telling me that my spine fracture was significant but would heal. He said I would go home in 2 days with lots of pain killers. "What!" I said, How on earth could I go home unable to move? From lying on the floor not wanting to be in hospital I now realised my condition was not something I wanted to monitor myself on the floor. As something is now seen to be broken, how long would it take to heal? I had broken my arm on 2 occasions in my life, I knew it takes weeks. Would I be on the floor in my house for weeks? How on earth would I eat, run a home with no movement and for how long?

By now there were enough blood pressure measurements to say there was something wrong with my heart that needed clarity. Again, I remember being wheeled this time remaining in the trauma bed, but wheeled for tests. Whoever would listen, I repeatedly said, *"There is nothing wrong with my heart. I do mindfulness, tai chi, qigong, I am a natural health therapist I practice slow for a living and a lifestyle, I do Nature Forest Therapy guided walks, I live in the slow lane. I value slow, I am happy my heart is slow, I am very healthy, just had an accident."* I felt I was talking to the walls.

I was being wheeled from one test to the next. Finally, I found myself, late at night, the hospital lights low, being wheeled out of a lift and met by a Cardiologist. *"Hello, my name is Dr Richardo… I am a Cardiologist."*

"I have nothing wrong with my heart. I don't know what they see on the charts, I value a slow heart, I work at being slow." Came my response.

"It's okay, I will give you a good report, you won't have to come to see us again, don't worry." replied Dr Richardo.

This was a different approach, I thought. Then being wheeled into a room another man, Andy from Taiwan, noticed the positioning of the previous electrodes on my chest saying, "they have put them in the wrong place, no wonder the results were not good. Don't worry."

From here there was a significant turning point. From fear and mistrust, feeling like I was an object, to a shift towards positivity. I was being cared for, I could feel the warmth and sensitivity as Andy put electrodes all over my chest, and with an ultrasound hand control with gel slowly moved the control around my upper body.

He moved the computer monitor where I could see it and said, *"Look, this is your heart. Now breathe while I take some photos. Breathing in, hold, wow, look how beautiful your heart is. I am going to look at it from multiple angles. Now see this, breathing in, hold… Oh look at this angle…Oh look at this view? It is so beautiful isn't it?."*

For what seemed like half an hour, I was given a tour of my heart finishing up with rivers of blue and red flowing in and out, being constantly told how amazing and beautiful my heart was.

That experience shifted my sense of where I was at in this experience. I now felt very clear where I was. I was in limbo in my body for sure, unable to move but in my heart, I was well, I was in a great place. And I knew exactly where I was going. If I can breathe then there is more right with me than wrong with me, said Jon Kabat Zinn, and now, not only can I breathe I have an amazing beautiful heart.

I fell off to sleep waking intermittently with the vision of the monitor and 'my beautiful heart'.

Here I am on Friday morning. The nurse has given me

pain killers, a needle to thin my blood, medication to make me go to the toilet as the pain killers cause constipation and nausea tablets to address the nausea from the medication, and oh yes, the acid tablets that address the acid that also results from the medication. From someone who took not even Panadol occasionally, I was now truly medicated.

I hadn't gone to the toilet and didn't feel an urge to go. I still couldn't move my back; the bed had a sit up lift but despite the pain medication I could not tolerate being moved. Eating and drinking was not possible, I could not sit up. Not being able to eat did not worry me. I decided to take water from time to time very carefully but not eating was okay for at least 2 days. Initially I was not hungry at all. The shock was very much in my stomach as well as my back. I felt nothing but tension in the trunk of my body.

I had been breathing, slowly and deeply with long out breaths since arriving in the hospital, and I was now working out what else I needed to do.

The first was to feel felt. As I started to notice softness and kindness, I was also acutely aware that I wanted to reach out to be kind to others too. How to be kind in such a vulnerable state. I said thank you as much as I could. As I started becoming curious, to connect to what was outside of me, I noticed the shock tailoring down. I did not want to talk on the phone, that would have taken me to explanations and reliving the pain.

No, I was very clear where I wanted my attention to be, I wanted to keep the positive energy of beauty and kindness as my life line and I needed to feel it in this reality, what was around me right in the here and now.

I looked out, in my line of sight to connect. I knew that fear, pain and worry would not be the conditions for healing to take place. And already I had the sense that it was not the policy of the hospital to nurture my natural healing. Some hospital staff may know how to do this, but I could see it was not a hospital policy. In the hours of my being in this position, as grateful as I was to have the pain killers and being in hospital care, I knew that I needed to find my own ways of nurturing my body's healing.

I could hear the conversation between the people in the room. People in their 80's spoke with distinct respect to each other. Listening in, I heard that one had spent his life as a journalist and the other as the wife of a musical agent being part of the 60' and 70's bringing artists from England to tour Australia. Their conversation engaged my social self, my sense of interest in another and wonder of curiosity in who, what, when and where.

I extended this sense of curiosity to the nurses, wondering where they came from, what lifestyles those countries had years ago when cultures were different from each other. I could feel kindness creeping towards me, softness and tenderness reaching across the spaces that were otherwise cold and distant.

Herbert Benson is a cardiologist, and founder of the Mind/Body Medical Institute at Massachusetts General Hospital in Boston. He is a professor of mind/body medicine at Harvard Medical School. In the late 1960's and through to the 1970's Dr Herbert Benson was one of the first academics to do research on the mind/body interaction, the impact the mind had on the body. His research began with transcendental meditation that was at the time being practiced by students at Harvard University. The meditators were excited at what they were experiencing, wanting to have some scientific perspective on what was happening.to them as they practiced meditating. At a time when the counter culture in the USA was inviting the east into the west, there were a scattering of academics who showed interest in scientifically researching how, 'mental focusing techniques were good for the body'.[1]

Herbert Benson was one of the first researchers to scientifically evaluate what effect, if at all, meditation now known as mindfulness has on the body. More recently he wrote:

> "Evolution has yielded us a human body that is astonishingly reliable, able to perpetuate breath and thought, movement and experience, day after day, year after year. By and large, our bodies function

even when we bombard them with stress and fatty food, even when we neglect to exercise or to get a good night's sleep. Clearly, we are blessed with an incredible internal technology....

Sadly though, we still rely far more than we should on external fixes – on medication and medical and surgical procedures developed in laboratories – and not on our natural potential for self-healing."[2]

As Herbert Benson explains,

"I envision a future in which medicine is as sturdy as a three-legged-stool, balanced equally by three healing resources – medications; surgery including other medical procedures; and self-care approaches.[3]"

Pills and procedures account for most modern medicine, in fact that is what I was experiencing in hospital, I could see that self-care was up to me. Herbert Benson even puts a ratio to the self-care percent of the three-legged-stool.

"Ideally medicine, would call upon self-care for 60 to 90 percent of the everyday problems that patients experience. We would draw appropriately upon the medicines and surgeries when necessary. All three legs are mandatory."[4]

Self-care for 60 to 90 percent of the patient experiences? That is not modern culture. How many times do people turn to medication for headaches, and pills for colds? If 60 to 90 percent of our medical experience could be dealt with by self-care, those practices are not well practiced by most of us. They are hidden from popular view. They are replaced by advertisements, commercial products and marketing of pills and procedures.

Self-care is not selfishness. Selfishness is when I care about myself and make sure that my needs are satisfied, regardless of others. Self-care on the other hand is when I care about self, not to the exclusion of considering others. On the contrary it would be within the interest of self-care to be considerate of others to reduce possible conflict, bad feelings or stress.

Self-care defined by the World Health Organisation is,'

> "the ability of individuals, families and communities to promote health, prevent disease, maintain health, and to cope with illness and disability with or without the support of a healthcare provider".

I was well aware that I had a task, how to apply self-care when unable to move. It was getting towards

Shabbat, Friday night where I would not have access to my phone for 25 hours. I explained to the nurse that I would not be using the buzzer and I would need to call out if I needed help. I thought carefully about how to use the next few hours before Shabbat came in.

I hadn't been to the toilet. I thought I should work out how that was going to happen while it was still daylight. I waited till I could feel the need to pass urine and I told the nurse. She pulled the curtain around which I realised would not create a wall of silence but rather a sense of privacy, and she brought a pan to the bed. She and another nurse very carefully rolled me over, positioned the pan and gently rolled me back. I actually was pleasantly surprised that this was actually possible and did not cause pain, but rather, slight discomfort which now the pain killers were blunting, but not pain. I relieved my bladder and with another roll, the pan was removed.

This was my first realisation of the sense of shame that comes with not being able to walk to the toilet and close the door. Over the next few days this shame became a key part of the hospital experience. We, the patients, all felt it in varying ways, our embarrassment, in my case to bring a bedpan, then remove it quickly, or in the case of my 'neighbours', help them to the toilet in time. The shame compounded when either the bedpan sat for some time not being removed, or with others, the relief of liquid or solid waste came before the nurse arrived.

I felt that we were all returning to babies, needing care givers to deal with our intimate needs of body fluids, and this need came with appreciation and also great shame. I looked enviously when a 'neighbour' made the trek to the toilet herself. It caused much cheering. I decided to drink sparingly and could manage another day without eating. I still had no hunger and although I was no longer cold and shivering, I had still a coldness internally, a sense of shut down that radiated throughout my body.

Fasting as an age-old practice, relates to religious rituals and holy days, to indigenous people's preparation to special celebration, meetings and gatherings, as well as attributed to cleaning the body for health benefits. I knew that fasting not only calmed down my nervous system but by doing so would enable more healing to occur during the night. I was very familiar with fasting and had for some time been aligning myself to the circadian rhythms.

In 2017 the Nobel Prize in Physiology or Medicine was awarded to Jeffrey C. Hall, Michael Rosbash and Michael W. Young for their discoveries of molecular mechanisms that control circadian rhythms. Like the birds, the trees, the flowers, the sea, the sun and the moon, there is a rhythm a natural timing in life.

Although Circadian rhythms have been known for centuries, every woman knows that menstruation has a cycle, and when women are living together, somehow that cycle becomes synchronised. We all know that the gestation time for babies in the womb is the same for all women. It may be more obvious in some places where seasons change the colour of the street, and where birds change their calls. However, for many people, now the rhythm of nature is outside of awareness, replaced by technology and empowered accessibility.

It is only recently, since the invention of electricity that night has become as light as the day and in the last 20 years with the phone and lap tops/iPad, that light has been accessible around the clock. For many people sleeping at night is interrupted by bright light whilst pursuing ideas, messages, work and pleasure and the impact this has is now being understood via the science of circadian rhythms.

The human disruption of our circadian rhythms has recently been identified as a critical part of disturbing the body's natural healing capacity. Circadian rhythms are controlled by what's known as circadian clocks. As Satchin Panda, one of the leading researchers in this new field of Circadian rhythm science says,

> "These (clocks) are actually encoded in our DNA. And this is so fundamental to life forms on our planet that if we move any animal or human from this planet to another planet that has identical conditions as the planet Earth but has a day-night cycle other than 24 hours then we cannot

easily survive. "[5]

Circadian rhythms are the code to health, Satchin Panda recounts. Each cell in our body functions according to rhythms that are clock driven.

> "..every organ has its own peak performance time at certain times of the day. And every organ needs to sleep, or rest and rejuvenate, at another time. So all these clocks work together to give us daily rhythms in sleep, metabolism, mood and even gut microbiome...
>
> ... Today, almost one-third of all adults suffer from at least one chronic disease, such as obesity, diabetes, cardiovascular disease, hypertension, respiratory disease, asthma, or chronic inflammation.... the truth about chronic disease is that there is rarely a cure. We just have better ways to manage and live with these diseases."[6]

Disrupting our circadian rhythms has now proven to increase the risk of several chronic diseases that are associated with aging.[7] All the cells in our body are designed for synchronicity as they each hold a variety of functions. To operate in well-being is for our body and brain cells to sleep, eat, fast and exercise according to the natural rhythms of the light/night sun cycle.[8]

The critical part of the scientific discovery of the circadian rhythms, is how our body operates as a whole connected system that directly relates to the rhythm of the natural light of day/night. Many studies were done with shift workers, who operate on their own sleep/work cycles and these all concluded towards the same direction of results, to the extent that in 2007 The World Health Organisation's International Agency for Research on Cancer classified shift work as a potential carcinogen.[9] As Satchin Panda points out,

> "if you stay awake for at least 3 hours between 10.00pm and 5.00am for more than 50 days a year, (once a week) you are a shift worker and at risk of suffering from shift-work related diseases."[10]

What is clear is that in today's world, we are all shift workers, because of the private and easy access we have to a life of 'day', at 'night'. It isn't enough to eat the right foods avoid the wrong foods and sleep so many hours. The 'when' is now seen as the critical part of health and the capacity for the body to fight off disease. Our cells throughout our body are designed to be in sync with the rhythm of healing and when this rhythm is disrupted the impact over time is disease.

Despite the introduction of artificial light in the last 100 years, it is the digital screens that have pushed us towards, what Satchin Panda calls, "a circadian collapse".

We are all aware with the feelings of moving from indoors to outside experiencing the natural light, especially on a sunny day and even more so, in the morning. It turns out that all of life, including us human beings, requires that our biology is tuned into the dawn and dusk for regulating all our bodily systems. Light effects our sight as much as light effects our internal cell clocks. The liminal times of sunrise and sunset are not just beautiful features of our world; They are designed as signals, gentle signals to get up and be active to walk and search for food as well as settle down to our last feed and wind down to sleep. The feeling to spring out of bed in the early morning, is a sign of good health just as the yawn and desire to sleep at night.

This rhythm is not just for convenience, it actually is the way our body systems can shift their multiple roles. Each cell in our body has multiple functioning. Cells need to distribute nutrients, clean out their dead cells or toxic waste, grow, develop and heal as well as send and receive messages. There is much that is still unknown regarding the function of our body cells. However, the discovery of the circadian rhythm mechanisms has unlocked a world of understanding in how and when our body heals itself naturally.

The circadian code as Satchin Panda calls it, includes natural light and the opposite, complete dark, moving the body in the morning and late afternoon as well as what he calls Time Restricted Eating. The time restricted eating relates to the when of our eating. These factors, the when of the light, the when of the exercise and the when of the eating as well as the when of sleeping either regulate or dysregulate our circadian rhythms. We feel it with jet lag and now the term 'social lag' is being used to describe that feeling out of sync with body and a foggy mind when we haven't slept all night. Babies develop their rhythms when they are about 3 months old, when we are lucky!

To the extent that sleeping at night, from 11.00 to 6.00 offers the signal of our body to switch on to its night work of healing our cells, the cells in our stomach cannot make this switch if it is busy digesting food. The extent to which our cells relate to the light and dark, our cells also relate to food and fasting. Food sets up, and it includes drink too, except plain water, a system of whole-body activation. From our salivary glands to our intestines preparing to operate, our body's pathway moves from a system of work with food, to a pathway of healing when our body is fasting. Time restricted eating is the term used to describe the circadian eating rhythm. It isn't about what you eat, you can eat whatever you like, although what you eat may have some impact on your nutrient intake. The real impact is the timing. According to Satchin Panda,

> "Time restricted eating is never about counting calories, it is just about making you more disciplined about timing. ..The moment you eat breakfast or have your first cup of tea or coffee is the beginning of your eating window. Once you set your breakfast time, stick with it. If breakfast begins at 8.00am, dinner must end of 8.00pm. ...at least 2 or 3 hours before your typical sleep time...This is important, as melatonin levels begin to rise 2 to 4 hours before your typical sleep time. Finishing your meals before melatonin begins to rise is necessary to escape the interfering effect of melatonin on blood sugar."[11]

Bone health is one of the specific areas that have been researched in relation to circadian rhythms, uncovering that there is a direct impact on circadian disruption and bone formation.[12]

> "..disruption of the circadian clock due to shift work, sleep restriction, or clock gene knockout is associated with osteoporosis or other abnormal bone metabolism, showing the importance of the circadian clock system for maintaining homeostasis of bone metabolism. Moreover, common

causes of osteoporosis, including postmenopausal status and aging, are associated with changes in the circadian clock".[13]

I had to wear a face mask upon entering the hospital and at some stage I asked the kind fellow with the green outfit if there was an eye mask I could wear in order to sleep. He said, 'Pull the face mask up over your face till it covers your eyes." Consequently, each night at around 8.00 pm, I put the face mask over my eyes. This was a critical part of my self-care. Avoiding the night electric lights.

CHAPTER 3

I had not eaten on the day and the following day of the accident and using the mask to cover my eyes at night was giving me a sense that my bones and muscles and whatever else was shutting down, turning off or broken, was being given time to heal. I was reminding myself of all the ways I can self-care. I was well aware that my nervous system was very much a key to protecting me from the trauma by shutting down, and I was conserving the little energy I had to be mindful. Firstly, mindful of breathing. I continuously turned by attention to noticing my breath, slow breaths that were longer on the out than on the in. Breathing into my pain, watching the rise and fall of the pain.

There was a young man opposite my bed who had shattered his elbow. He owned a bar and was renovating it. While he was checking out the latest changes, he fell over something. It was late when he arrived at the hospital. It was the middle of the night when he returned from the surgery. He was very upset, yelling out that there was not enough pain relief. He was finding it hard to wait for his next medication and so I called out to him, "breathe into your pain, welcome it as you would a friend who is hurt, and breathe into it. Slow breath in and even slower breath out. Imagine your inhale entering into this pain, holding it with your breath and as you breathe out slowly see it reduce in size and in depth." From across the aisle, I breathed with him, and eventually I heard him go off to sleep. It didn't last for too long, but long enough to reaffirm that by helping him and seeing the difference it made for his pain, I was encouraging my healing too. I was reinforcing my healing attitude.

Most people are familiar with a smile leading to a smile, a laugh inviting others to laugh and a sigh or yawn tempting further sighs and yawns. These behaviours are known as emotional or social contagions, a term that explains the system of mirror neurons that are inbuilt in our biology for social engagement, learning and perceiving intention.

Dan Siegal the founder of Interpersonal Neurobiology offers an insight into how this works. He calls these mirror neurons, 'sponge neurons',[1] as they soak up what you see in someone else. The energy field that is within your body flows and is met by my energy field and this he calls 'information energy flow'. Our bodies and mind combine to send cues and signals to each other. If someone waves their hands around, or repeatedly taps a finger, this does not activate my mirror neurons, it does not signal to me that I wish to do the same behaviour. However, mindful breathing, yawning, sighing, laughing and drinking water or eating food in front of me activates a linking map in my head that forms a connection between seeing and doing. The information that is being sent to me activates a knowing in my body that reacts by doing what I am seeing. By my breathing slowly and exhaling longer than inhaling, across the room as well as sending words and information towards my 'neighbour,' mirror neurons were picking up the signals of tranquility and thus able to entrain him to calm.

Breath in Hebrew is the same word for spirit. We all know that the breath is the first and last state of life. Its role in regulating our mind and body is complex. In an article published in 2018, looking at the role of breath in the body, the authors conclude:

> 'In its contractions, the diaphragm muscle has systemic functional reflexes that are not only related to changes in tissue oxygen. In this article, we reviewed some functions not yet well explored, such as the neural oscillations, the movement of the brain

> mass, the influences that the breath has on motor activities, and the electrical responses of the brain at low voltage (the latter through variations of blood intracranial pressures). The diaphragm still has many mysteries to be unveiled, not only on the functions it exerts in the body system but also on the usefulness that a manual approach can have on the patient…..
>
> … Breath has patterns. Schemes create behavior. Breath is a behavior. Behavior represents the person. Breath reveals the person."[2]

James Nestor, journalist and author of the Breath, the New Science of The Lost Art, uses his personal experience of asthma to begin a journey of enquiry that led him on a 10-year exploration through not only the scientific understandings of breathing but the cultural diversity of how breathe was and still is used as a healing art. In responding to questions in 2020 he explains:

> "Evolution does not mean survival of the fittest. Evolution means change. And life forms can change for the better or the worst. Humans today have been changing in many ways that are of no benefit to long term health. Especially in consideration to our breathing…

> ...When we take in air (through our noses) we force air through this labyrinth (of sinus pathways) until it reaches our throats then goes into our lungs. The reason is, we want air to be conditioned, heated, moistened and pressurised before it reaches our lungs. And that is exactly what the nose and the sinuses do. When we breathe through the mouth, we get none of those benefits. You get 20% more oxygen in each nasal breath than you do with a breath through the mouth...
>
> .. By breathing, always through the nose, slowly and breathing less, you increase circulation, increase oxygenation, you can significantly lower your blood pressure and you can allow the systems of your body to work in harmony with one another. That is why this breathing pattern, this 5 to 6 seconds in and 5 to 6 seconds out has been found to be so effective... you are allowing your body to heal itself; you are allowing your body to do more with less effort.".[3]

When we are under stress, our breathing patterns change.

In 1915, Walter B. Cannon whilst a professor in Physiology at Harvard University coined the term 'Fight or Flight' response to describe an animal's response to threats in bodily changes in pain, hunger, fear and rage.[4] Years later it was Hans Selye's research as Physician and Endocrinologist that took him to use the term 'stress response' to describe the body's natural reaction to adverse events. As a 2nd year student in the University of Prague Medical school where the approach then in the 1920's,, and still exists today within the medical profession, requires investigating for signs, symptoms and factors that are particular to certain illnesses, Hans Selye noticed something else amongst all the patients. What Hans Selye noticed was, the patients had a common theme, such as looking tired, having no appetite, losing weight, preferring to lie down rather than stand, and not being in the mood to go to work. He called it the *"syndrome of just being sick"*[5]. It took him years later to give a clear understanding of the physiological pathway that would link what hadn't really been linked before. That is that there is a general reaction to the body, to all forms of stress. We see that today, the term stress is universally used to describe not only the physiological or pathological domain, but also within the context of economical, philosophical and social factors that contribute to individuals and society.[6]

Herbert Benson in the same laboratory that Walter Cannon used for his fight/flight research in the early 1920s, found the opposite is also true, that to the extent the body reacts to stress by releasing hormones that increase heart rate, speeding up blood flow to the muscles getting us ready to fight or flight, so the opposite holds true.

> "The body is also imbued with what I termed the Relaxation Response. – an inducible physiologic state of quietude. Indeed, our progenitors handed down to us a second, equally essential survival mechanism - the ability to heal and rejuvenate our bodies. In modern times, the Relaxation Response is undoubtedly even more important to our survival, since anxiety and tension often inappropriately trigger the fight-or-flight response in us. Regular elicitation of the Relaxation Response can prevent, and compensate for, the damage incurred by frequent nervous reactions that pulse through our hearts and bodies."[7]

The connection between the mind and body is symbiotic. One impacts on the other. I was sure that my body's energy system was blocked from the trauma and I wanted to find a way of signaling to my body that it can relax now, it is safe.

Strange as it may seem, talking to my body, I knew from years of working with alternative therapies as a professional as well as my personal practices, that communication lies at the heart of healing. Not necessarily out loud verbal communication, but messages sent and received create the spectrum between harm and healing. Now, lying in bed, unable to lift my head or body, I had a busy time ahead of me planning how I could reach the cells in my mind and body to heal.

Most people are familiar with the placebo effect, but not many are aware of the opposite, the nocebo. Associate Professor in the Faculty of Science and Leader of the Placebo Research Network at the Charles Perkins Centre at the University of Sydney, has developed a number of novel experimental models to uncover the mechanisms of placebo and nocebo effects for pain, sleep, nausea, and related conditions.

> "We're finding that the main way placebos work, is to influence the person's expectations, or their mindset, which then affects how their body reacts," says Colagiuri.[8]

In an interview published in the Australian Pain Society in 2019 about his research in both placebo and nocebo he said:

> "An early negative experience in a clinic could set you up for a long-term nocebo effect." [9]

I knew that the sooner I got into a rhythm of healing the better chance I was going to give my body. The rhythm needed to be within my body, a coherent connection between my feelings, thinking and body. The research of the past 10 years through the sports science industry has made this connection to be the difference between the number one winner and the rest.[10] As Dr David Hamilton, former scientist from within the pharmaceutical industry points out, there has been an exponential growth in the amount of interest, academically in scientific journals, in the past few years in areas called visualisation, mental practice, mental imagery, guided imagery, motor imagery and kinaesthetic imagery. All these terms to describe the use of mind in relation to the body. This research is mainly in the areas of sports and rehabilitation. Before we take a look at this recent research development let us go back to the beginning of the field of medicine, back to the 16th and 17th century.

The separation between the body and the experiences that go in inside the body named as feeling or emotional states has been part of western thinking since the acceptance of Rene Descartes, in the 17th century. The idea that mind and body are really distinct—a thesis now called "mind-body dualism," lies at the heart of our medical professionals teaching. In an article titled Mind-body Dualism: A critique from a Health Perspective,[11] Neeta Mehta, Associate Professor from the Department of Psychology, V.G. Vaze College (affiliated to Mumbai University), writes:

> "....The field, which is facing crisis today, is that of medicine, and the paradigmatic stance that is responsible for the crisis is Cartesian dualism—a view that mind and body are essentially separate entities...
>
> ...Mind and body dualism was the critical conceptual leap that was desperately sought at that time in history. Before its

advent, the prevalent orthodox Christian views of the mind-body relationship had greatly thwarted the development of medical science. According to these views, human beings were spiritual beings; body and soul were one. Diseases were attributed to nonmaterial forces such as personal/collective wrongdoing. It was also believed that for the soul to ascend to heaven, the human body had to be preserved intact. As a result, there was a religious prohibition on the study of human anatomy through dissection. Descartes, through mind-body dualism, demythologised body and handed over its study to medicine. Thus, the way was paved for progress in medical science through the study of physiology and anatomy. At the same time, by isolating mind, mind and body dualism denied its significance in individuals' experience of health."[12]

As Neeta Mehta concludes in her paper,

"Mind-body dualism is an example of a metaphysical stance that was once much needed to unshackle science and medicine from dogma, but which later had far reaching restrictive influence on the field of medicine, on its complete understanding of real health issues, and on developing effective interventions to deal with the same."[13]

Self-Care the real story of healing

The framework of mind body has a cultural history. Despite many health professionals especially in the complimentary medicine field, encouraging mind body connection; there is resistance that is heavily guarded, to separate the two. Neeta Mehta points out the philosophy behind medical practice lies behind the scenes whether one is aware or not.

This philosophy has impact not only on the research and development of the learning in medicine but more importantly on the way medicine is practiced, by professional or patient. If mind-body is seen as separate, then as a patient or as a professional we are processing information very differently than if we see life, all of life as interconnected. This then, the interconnected mind body theory is where the holistic health perspective draws its practices from.

Barbara Fredrickson, the Kenan Distinguished Professor of Psychology at the University of North Carolina at Chapel Hill, is well known for her 'broaden and build theory', developed in 1998. She recognises that whilst negative emotions narrow thought-action repertoires, positive emotions broaden thought-action repertoires.[14] Later in 2013 her book titled Love 2.0 Finding Happiness and Health in Moments of Connection, further elaborates on the embodiment of emotions.

> "For just as neuroscientific studies show that positive emotions open your perceptual awareness, kinematic studies ... show that they also open your torso, literally expanding the (rib) cage in which

your heart sits. When your mind and body are infused with good feelings, those feelings lift and expand your chest, a subtle nonverbal gesture that makes you more inviting to others, more open for connection."[15]

Embodiment is defined as having, being in, or being associated with a body. There is a whole field now in psychology called Somatic Psychotherapy that is body centred psychotherapy. Here. the therapeutic approach is designed to integrate the physical body into the therapy process.

Returning to research done on rehabilitation and mental imagery, (body and mind connection), the use of visualisation to aid rehabilitation needed to be in addition to movement:

"Visualisation is not a substitute for medical advice, but something that we use in addition to medical advice. .. No matter what therapy or drugs a person receives for an injury or medical condition, they have to think. That's the nature of the mind. The mind will wander in one direction or the another. While wandering towards stressful thoughts might not be helpful, when the mind is focused in a positive way the benefits can be positive. In effect, visualization guides us in the *content* of our thinking, targeting it in a positive constructive way. But in a way that we're learning also has direct effects of its own, beyond simply sparing us some stress."[16]

I knew that although it was only my back that was broken, the trauma I had experienced was reverberating all over me including my mind. On this second night in hospital, in the room I would stay in for almost 2 weeks, I prepared some healing strategies. One of the latest modalities I was practicing and continuing to learn, was a body therapy.

Ortho-Bionomy was developed in the late 1970's by Arthur Linus Paul. Originally Canadian, he was a martial art teacher in England and a student of Osteopathy. Lawrence Jones, an osteopathic teacher taught and wrote of the spontaneous release by positioning.[17] Arthur Pauls took this direction and extended it to include a holistic approach and integrating modality, drawing on his knowledge and experience of martial arts and homeopathy. The focus in Ortho-Bionomy is no pain to reduce pain. Attention is given to where pain trigger points are found, and with gentle positioning and other techniques, pain is reduced. The work includes energy releasing and balancing where the practitioner does not use body positioning but rather a hands-off approach focusing on what is known in the martial arts world as energy fields.

Having studied natural therapies over 30 years ago and energetic healing being part of my practice, it was easy to see that Ortho-Bionomy is an integrated training bringing the knowledge of east and west, mind and body, together.

Dr. Colin A. Ross. Psychiatrist, is the Director of hospital-based Trauma Programs in Denton, Texas, Torrance, California and Grand Rapids, Michigan. In his book, Human Energy Fields, he says that energy fields that are called *chi*, the human aura, the life force, or the human spirit in different philosophical systems; and the scientific term known as electromagnetic field of the body, are the same thing.[18] Different cultural terms for describing the same phenomena.

I had been studying Tai Chi for the past few years and noticed the significant impact that this practice had on my body and mind. The slow movements had both internal feelings as well as noticing the external elements. Slowing down movement brings conscious awareness to not just the body but the air around. In a paper titled Connecting Western and Eastern Medicine from an Energy Perspective, the authors look towards common themes such as opposing forces, and the balance of these forces which create homeostasis otherwise known as balance.

> " Although Western medicine and Eastern medicine are worlds apart, there is a striking overlap in the basic principle of these types of medicine when we look at them from the perspective of energy. In both worlds, opposing forces provide the energy that flows through networks in an organism, which fuels life. In this concept, health is the ability of an organism to maintain the balance between these opposing forces, i.e., homeostasis (West)

> and harmony (East), which creates resilience….
>
> ….Health can be defined as the ability to adapt to challenges. When we have stress, a challenge, there is an attack on our energy. The energy goes down, but our body has resilience to absorb the challenge and bounce back. In the rebound, there is even a temporary improvement and you build up resistance. Thus, a little bit of bad is good for you, ..We do have a problem when the challenge is intense and prolonged. For example, due to a chronic illness, the energy decreases and reaches a new equilibrium at a lower energy level. In this condition, we can no longer cope with even a small challenge. All energy might flow away and then it is the end."[19]

Western medicine uses pills to change the molecular pattern of energy in the body. In the east, a more intuitive approach is used. Despite the lack of science behind intuitive approaches, research on tai chi, qigong and acupuncture[20] reveal a very strong acceptance now amongst many western people including doctors and scientists.

I added a few more strategies for healing. Drawing on the self-care of Ortho-Bionomy, I visualised my bones, muscles, connective tissues, nervous system and fluids, healing and balancing from my head to my feet. I would often stray from this focus, but I had nothing else to do, no need to hurry, or be annoyed because I got lost in thoughts. I just came back to where I left off, and continued till I had summoned these parts, systems of my body to healing. I then googled tai chi lying in bed, and found a video of a 25 minute guided qigong practice for lying down. This was amazing. Although I could not move much, I practiced the visualising and the qigong 3 times a day and each time, noticed more movement.

The most astonishing experience I discovered in doing the qigong was the energy awareness. I could feel the block of energy the stuckness of my body and as I slowly moved my hands, I could feel the flow of energy moving. Almost like a soft breeze I could feel the air move and with it my internal body mirror the flow.

Visualising walking along the beach, swimming and the feeling of the ground under by feet, was a key part of my program. I would imagine the slow walks, even imaging the wind, smelling the sea air, feeling the cold, or the wet of the water when I imagined swimming. I used the visualising along with the breathing. Breathing in and feeling my body expand, putting attention on the pain areas and breathing out imagining the inflammation reduce, the pain getting smaller. Deep slow gentle breaths of in expand, out, reduce.

Saturday night after sunset I put my phone back on, and looked for 'stand-up comedy on corona'. I found a few videos and spent 2 hours laughing at the comedy. I am sure the other people including the nurses thought I was quite crazy, but I knew that laughter increased my natural endorphins and that night I did not need the midnight pain killers. This was the beginning of my pain killer reduction.

> "Relaxed social (Duchenne) laughter is associated with feelings of wellbeing and heightened affect, a proximate explanation for which might be the release of endorphins. We tested this hypothesis in a series of six experimental studies in both the laboratory (watching videos) and naturalistic contexts (watching stage performances), using change in pain threshold as an assay for endorphin release. The results show that pain thresholds are significantly higher after laughter than in the control condition." [21]

I was now ready to eat, not much, but I found I could lift my head slightly more and although I had no appetite, I wanted to enjoy something. One of the nurses had said to me, "eat what you like to eat, it is important to get your appetite going." There was a banana next to me, and boy, did I enjoy that banana.

I also noticed my stomach was very tight. I was taking medication to relieve my bowels but so far nothing had been released. I tried some shiatsu on myself. Pressing down on pressure points in a circular motion in a particular order released the tightness in my stomach and intestinal area and again, I could feel the energy begin to untangle. Between the qigong, the laughter and the visualisations, I was very busy. On Monday morning a neurosurgeon doctor arrived, not the one that I had seen in emergency. This doctor told me that the physio therapist would see me soon, and get me to sit up. This I found hard to believe. There is a large gap between someone telling you to do something that feels is way out of depth, and telling yourself though visualisation what you can do. One way is power over and the other is power within. I knew that I still couldn't sit up. I could feel recovery in process but I also could see they were minute shifts. In fact when I asked the nurse to look at how much I could do now, I saw the look on her face of " no, I can't see any difference.".

When the physio therapist came, I told her what had happened, how I was traumatised by sitting on the chair in my home, and could not raise myself or have the bed raised as the pain was unbearable. The physio heard what I said, but repeated that they, there were 2 of them, would lift me to sit up. She said, "you are safe", which did not resonate with me at all.

The word safe carries enormous meaning. To the extent that danger signals the body to go into fight or flight, safeness signals the body to relax and be calm. Telling someone they are safe is not the signal. The signal is a felt sense, not a signpost. We see signs in our urban word "Danger" often, at building sites, along footpaths, at gates that have dogs behind them. These words by themselves do not signal the body to jump or run away. On the contrary, they tell us not to go there, from a cognitive moral understanding. A child who cannot read will not obey the words, unless they come with a felt experience of knowing. The actual experience of dogs barking or the smell of fire or falling into a hole, these experiences are what take us to fight/flight. I understood that the purpose of telling me I was safe was to encourage my felt sense of safeness. However, the word itself without any safe feeling connected to it held no impact on me at all. As Dr Paul Gilbert says, safety is different from safeness. A seat belt is a safety feature, safeness however is the feeling that being in bed on a cold night, with a hot water bottle, bed socks and being tucked in, creates in your whole body.

Dr Paul Gilbert has developed Compassion Focused Therapy is the Professor of Clinical Psychology at the University of Derby and Visiting Professor at the University of Queensland. One of the key concepts in his model of Compassion Focused Therapy is the three emotional regulation systems. When these are balanced, they offer us resources for survival, as well as thriving and wellbeing.

At the base of the model is the threat system. The system that is cued by danger. This cue sends the body to fight or flight, shutting down all the other body functions that are not required, enabling the body to harness all the power needed for self-protection.

The drive system is cued by wanting or striving. It induces us towards goals, focusing our attention on pursuing something. This is a double-edged sword. On the one hand this can lead to action for well-being, whilst on the other hand the expectation for the hormonal release of dopamine can take us to addiction.

The third regulatory system is the caring system. This is related to the gentle side of ourselves, the nurturing, place of safeness. The part of our body, mind and heart that is cued from kindness.[22] Paul Gilbert shows us the complexity of the interaction between safeness and threat in this diagram[23]. Safeness requires the cues that are felt from the body, as the body has its own surveillance system. With the cue of safeness there is a suppression of threat/defend hormones, with the absence of safeness there is a release of threat/defend hormones. Automatically our curiosity, play and capacity to discover are either turned up or turned off, based on our sense of feeling safe.

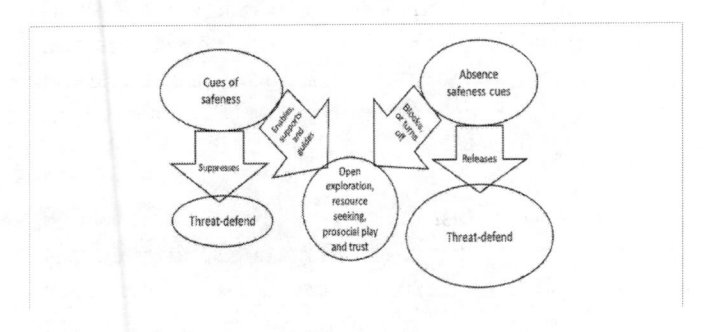

Stephen Porges, Distinguished University Scientist, at the Kinsey Institute, Indiana University Bloomington and professor in the department of psychiatry at the University of North Carolina in Chapel Hill in North Carolina, developed the Polyvagal Theory to describe how the autonomic nervous system is regulated by our external as well as our internal world. At the heart of his explanation is that we are designed as a surveillance system.[24]

Self-Care the real story of healing

> "These autonomic subsystems are phylogenetically ordered and behaviourally linked to social communication (e.g., facial expression, vocalization, listening), mobilization (e.g., fight–flight behaviours), and immobilization (e.g., feigning death, vasovagal syncope, and behavioural shutdown)."[25]

The trauma of my accident cued my body for danger, I was very much locked down from the pain and suffering, and the strategies in my self-care toolbox were guiding my body to feel safe, slowly and with consideration to the physical reality of a broken back. The kindness from the nurses, the others in the room, and the gratitude I had for being in a place where I could just put my attention on healing, was a key part of my recovery.

The physio therapist telling me I was safe, whilst lifting me in a position that I feared was not, did not contribute to cuing my body for safety. I had seen how quickly people were sent home. Over the weekend I had heard how the physios made the key decisions around staying in the hospital, going to rehabilitation or going home. I knew my recovery needed to be in hospital without being rushed, with time to heal along with the support of the hospital and my self-care strategies. I felt I needed to respect the physio therapist whilst at the same time respect my own knowledge. Mmm, what to do.

With much trepidation, I allowed them to put their hands under my arms and 1, 2, 3…..despite the pain killers, I could feel the shudder of agony, of ripples of pain shooting up my back into spasms. I was able to call out, and insist I go down. The sense of relief in being flat was immediate. I could see the physio therapist was not happy with me, and actually the feeling was mutual, I apologised, and said "thank you, I now know what to work on." In my mind I created a title for the physios. It made me laugh. I called them trauma specialists. Specialising in giving trauma.

CHAPTER 4

I was pleased the physio therapists left me alone, and I wondered how to proceed. I knew I could not trust them with my recovery, at least not these ladies. The following day was Sukkot, a Jewish holy day that is celebrated by eating all our meals in temporary huts. Of course, for me being in the hospital, it would not be possible, but the emotion of this holy day was one of happiness, of joy. This I could celebrate. I rang my friend and asked her to check with her husband, the Rabbi of the synagogue I attended, if due to the Jewish holy day, I could not have the physio for the next 2 days. The feedback was *"Yes, you should avoid doing anything that will interfere with your joy on these 2 days."*

One of the health benefits of being a religious Jew is the holy days. Every Friday night till Saturday night, we make Shabbat, A time where all technology is put aside, no car, no use of electricity, no work. All cooking is done by sunset Friday and the Shabbat is spent in the joy of experiencing life on a spiritual level rather than the usual mundane level. Experiencing life on the spiritual level is of course very hard to do given we have physical bodies and live in a material world. In order to experience this heightened sense of extraordinariness, it is the things we don't engage in, the usual routine of daily life that we avoid, that can support our directed attention. Just as the holy day of Yom Kippur was to take us to the emotional awareness of broken relationships between us and fellow human beings as well as our disconnection from our creator, so Sukkot is the festival of joy being reunified with our creator as well as our fellow human beings. The hut is symbolic of the temporary nature of life. That all things come and go, that just as a temporary hut is vulnerable to the weather, we are reminded by eating all our meals in it over the 7 days of Sukkot, that we too are vulnerable to nature, our human nature as well as the nature around us. The hut has specific requirements of measurement that include continuous walls as well as openings. This has the feeling, when you are inside the temporary dwelling, that you are being hugged. Sukkot is a festival that is inclusive of all people, it is symbolic of being at one with our creator and our fellow creatures, in joy.

For many people the concept of a creator is mythical. Something that modern day science discards as old fashioned. Today, evolutionary science is the bedrock of many explanations of where we and the rest of the world come from, and although evolutionary theory and the theory of a creator do not cancel each other out, there is often a sense that they are not equally respected in our modern culture. Whilst indigenous people all over the world see nature as a web of connectedness that humans are part of, they also see

Self-Care the real story of healing

this web includes spiritual energy that is unlimited. It is this unlimited energy that brings forth life. The source of life force. For people who believe in the creator, there is a power that comes with being connected to this source of life. In Judaism this power is seen to be in partnership with us.

Now how was I going to change my body in 2 days. I wanted to be able to sit without pain by Thursday morning. That would be 1 week from my accident. I knew I was making good progress but I needed to increase the pace. I included another affirmation to my routine. By tuning into my nervous system and thanking it for shutting down to avoid further damage to my spine, I was encouraging my nervous system to relax. It no longer needed to be cued for danger. It could know that I would not sit up until 'it' is ready. Although I was imagining a relaxed response in my nervous system and the muscles in my back, I did not feel this would be enough. I needed to bring out the Ace of all dreams. I prayed to g-d to heal my back so Thursday I could sit without the pain and without the fear of the physios.

Prayer is a form of communication. Ever since I can remember I have used language, quiet deep questions, plea's, statements and gratitude towards a sense of a good power that reaches out to beyond as well as inward, deep within my being. I can recall moments of deep pain, as a child listening to my parents fighting. Not hearing their words but feeling their intensity shatter my world. I would place my pillow over my ears to block out the sounds, and would wish they would stop. I didn't understand much about life, about the future or what can or can't happen. But I did know deep inside what pain was and that it is temporary, it comes and it goes. There were times when fighting didn't happen. In bed, as a 3-year-old or as a 63 year old, it was easy to go deep inside and pray.

When I started my religious journey, I was given a book of tehilim, the book of King David's psalms. It was a surprise to read the pain that the poetry explored, more than a hundred poems that spoke of deep anger, fear, jealousy, gratitude and hope. The surprise was the power of emotional connection, stories that sang the vibrations of life's inner world. Suffering, and the expression of suffering alongside not being alone in this, creates space for hope, for otherness besides suffering, to come. I knew that the formal religious idea of prayer was not the only way prayer has power.

Over 40 years ago I had travelled and lived in many countries around the world. In Japan I was intrigued, as most people are, with the traditional culture that is embedded in the modern city of Tokyo. Alongside the state of the art technological and computer era were temples that were full of people, local people kneeling, clapping, sitting in silence on pillows and off pillows. These temples were Buddhist and Shinto, religions that did not come from Judaism as Christianity and Islam did. They did not have the stories of floods or miracles that lay the foundation to the Abrahamic faiths. Despite the different beginning, Buddhism and Shintoism included practices and ways of directing attention towards respecting an invisible, indescribable power. A power that required reverence in order to get to a place of peace. This respect was directed to nature as well as beyond nature. The force was within man as well outside human form. The many Japanese traditional arts, such as flower arranging, tea ceremony, aikido, kendo and even wearing kimono have their essence in reverence, respect, harmony and zen.

Zen is a form of Japanese Buddhism which does not limit itself to sitting on a cushion but is found in every aspect of living. Zen refers to 'not one not two". A sense that there is a movement in life that does not reside in separateness. The idea that I am me, separate to you, is from a zen point of view missing the reality that I only exist because of the air that comes through me, the dependent arising of existence. That air also is going through you. Nothing is separate because life requires many conditions to exist. So 'not two' refers to not being dualist, that separateness, two, does not truly exist. 'Not one' refers to the notion that all is unity, the sense one gets when in the space of transcending the duality that happens in deep meditation. That sense of not one, that I do not feel myself, rather I have become one with the ocean of life. No longer a water droplet. 'Not one', is also transitory and so cannot be the true identity.

Hence as if we see walking as a metaphor, we walk with two feet and the balance that is seen and felt from rhythmic walking, requires an inbetweenness of not one foot on the ground, and not two feet on the ground, we actually balance from a betweenness of rhythm and awareness of this rhythm.

> "The free, bilateral movement between "not one" and "not two" characterizes

> Zen's achievement of a personhood with a *third* perspective that cannot, however, be confined to either dualism or non-dualism, neither "not one" nor "not two".[1]

This notion of seeing the world as not separate and yet not unified and yet both, includes then an acceptance of spiritual reality. The Japanese traditional arts, were a way of embodying this through 'kata', or particular form. For example, in the Japanese tea ceremony the kata would be found in the way one sits, gives, receives, picks up and puts down. Initially these forms are repeated and refined until there is a flow that embodies this rhythm of reverence, respect, awareness of not one, not two in my movements, attitude and attention. In Tai Chi it took me a long time to learn the form which is a choreograph of feet and hand movements that although very specific are also relaxed in the body.

A Chinese young man once told me, the most important part in the practice of Tai Chi is to feel the air outside and the flow of that air inside. All the Japanese arts include a form that creates this flow between the body and the object or art. It is very noticeable in watching the grace that comes with martial arts, the way of harnessing the energy that flows between the body and the space it is inhabiting. This form of attention creates a physical discipline of mindfulness, of space that allows for attention to be focused in a soft way. To the extent that prayer is about talking, mindfulness is about listening.

Connecting to the creator, for me, has meant to listen as well as to speak.

Self-Care the real story of healing

I added the affirmation: "Every day, in every way, I am getting better and better." This was something my memory connected to from the 1970's. Affirmations were part of the alternative therapy movement. Louise Hay had made this popular in my time, although the exact phrase is said to have been the words of Emile Coue, a French Pharmacist who graduated in 1876.

> "The Coué method centered on a routine repetition of this particular expression according to a specified ritual—preferably as many as twenty times a day, and especially at the beginning and at the end of each day. When asked whether or not he thought of himself as a healer, Coué often stated that "I have never cured anyone in my life. All I do is show people how they can cure themselves." Unlike a commonly held belief that a strong conscious will constitutes the best path to success, Coué maintained that curing some of our troubles requires a change in our unconscious thought, which can be achieved only by using our imagination."[2]

I had two days ahead for intense self-care. The nurse from Nepal was on duty looking after me this morning, she was very soft and kind. She certainly put me into a safeness place. She gave me a sponge bath in bed and changed the sheets, with my slight rolls to the right and to the left, my body as well as my mind was moving yet into another level of calm. In many ways being in this shutdown place of no movement brought me to connect with flowers and trees. The way I notice the sun and rain impacting on the earth, was how I was experiencing life now. Not being free to get up and go, I was subject to what was happening around me and to me. With the soft and gentle attention, the cells in my body were waking up, I could sense a shift in vibrations.

Empowerment now was not about taking myself to the toilet or going for a swim, or even being able to reach for a book. Empowerment was now being experienced in where would I put my attention. A new pattern for days emerged. Wake up to the sun, prayers of gratitude for being alive and connecting with the source of life with thanks for a new day. If the nurse didn't open the curtain, I would ask for it. Then my visualisations: calling on bones, muscles, connective tissues, nervous system and finally the liquids to be healed and well. Lying down tai chi/qigong followed by breathing. I had started eating fruit at 9.00am, kosher vegetarian lunch when it came, which was delicious. No dinner, as I was hardly moving and was keeping the circadian rhythms as the framework for the day. The pain medication was now working well and with the laughter at night, I had begun reducing the amount of *endone,* opioid pain-relief medicine, and this supported my intuition that my body was healing. Once I finished the morning routine, I was interested in what was happening around me.

The lady, Betty, next to me had snored the first night I had been up in this ward and I was very disturbed that I wouldn't be able to sleep, especially knowing how important the night sleeps are to body healing. Once I realised that was not going to change, neither her nor I were moving, I shifted my attitude and made peace with the reality. I started making more conversation and by this time we had created quite a nice feeling in the room. Robert, the journalist was very entertaining, telling us stories of his professional highlights and the changes over the years in the news reporting industry. We took turns in sharing stories that made us laugh or took us to interesting places, from our beds we were going back in time to before the 2nd world war, when Australia was wilder than it is today, the sand dunes of Maroubra and Bondi have since become urban hubs. We visited parties in England that were held by a river with activities such as fishing, lawn bowls and music with visitors such as the Prince of Wales attended. We heard how D.H. Lawrences' book Kangaroo, was actually based on true events at the time when D. H. Lawrence was in Australia. The laughter sessions were making me very light and easy to see the funny side of things.

We all had physical limitations, obviously that is why we were in hospital and now we had become more than patients sharing a ward, more like brothers and sisters sharing a bedroom. It was so interesting having such intimacy with strangers, and rather than shunning from the closeness, we started to accept it and be curious of each other's lives.

The fellow with the shattered elbow had gone and was replaced with different people who came and went. I noticed that no staff, doctors, nurses or physios went beyond the pills and procedures of medicine. I didn't witness self-care as part of the hospital system, I could see it was not part of our shared cultural knowledge or practice. Physio therapists came to take those who couldn't walk alone, for short walks. Due to lockdown, we had no visitors, only the hospital staff and each other.

At one stage a young lady was admitted to our room and she had something that took all her muscles away from their functional practice, leaving her bit by bit unable to even pick up a bottle of water without it going flying. Her walk, grip and movements, she said, were disconnected from her mindpower. She had been moved from a hospital that had no doctors who could work with this condition as it was stress related, with no physical justification except that she had no control over her movements. I asked her if it she had been traumatised, very stressed. She went on to describe her full-time study, full time work, divorce her parents had recently informed her of, the death of a close friend and how she found it hard to say no when people needed help. Perhaps lockdown had taken her past her point of coping, I don't know. It was so sad to see someone so young in such a state and I knew the longer her muscles forget about their networks the harder recovery may be. What you don't use you lose.

Gabor Mate is a Hungarian-Canadian physician and author of "When The Body Says No; The Cost of Hidden Stress." He brings his life experience, work as a family physician as well his scientific knowledge and insight into addiction, to bring out the body mind relationship of trauma. In a utube video, Gabor Mate says,

> "Trauma is not what happens to you, it is what happens inside of you. That's a good

thing by the way. Because if trauma, in terms of what happened to me as a Jewish infant under the Nazi's, if that was the trauma, I'll never be a person who wasn't a Jewish person under the Nazis, and during that period of genocide, …

..If trauma happened inside of you, the wound you sustained, the meaning you made of it, the way you then came to believe certain things about yourself, or the world or other people, and if trauma was that disconnection from your authentic self, well guess what. Good news! That can be restored at any moment…

.. when we see trauma as that wound, as long as we see it that way, it is a wound that can be healed. If we see it as a bunch of things that happened, that will never unhappen."[3]

The trauma of breaking my back was not just a physical experience, the loss of control I was experiencing in my physical world was being experienced in who I am, how I am being seen, my very identity is changing and this then is affecting my role in life. I am not just a mind and not just a body, they are connected and interdependent and include my social self. What I am experiencing in hospital in this condition is a realisation that my life has been largely about my social self, the part that interacts, engages in the give and take with others. Without the social self being active and empowered with busyness, I placed my attention on healing my body. I was recreating my sense of identity.

I was experiencing a very different social self, as well as physical and mental self. The me who was defined via the power to move was now being replaced by the me who had to deal with humiliation and the kindness of others to have all my physical needs met. This was a different experience of life.

After 20 years of family practice and palliative care experience, Dr. Gabor Maté worked for over a decade in Vancouver's Downtown East Side with patients challenged by drug addiction and mental illness. Author of many books that draw on science as well as his experience as a medical doctor, it is evident that he saw being a doctor as much more that a body physician, he connected with the person who came before him, not just the physical that could be poked and tested, but the complex person who was inhabiting the body. Through his awareness of the power of stress and the continuous interest he took of his patients lives, he came to see what Hans Selye saw, that the stress connection which in repeated and or extreme cases is more like trauma, lay behind disease. Not just the wounds from what happened but also for many people the human needs for love and kindness that did not happen.

> "The emotions and physical sensations that were imprinted during the trauma are experienced not as memories but as disruptive physical reactions in the present."[4]

Self-Care the real story of healing

Bessel Van Der Kolk, is one of the leaders in the trauma recovery field. Born in Holland he had his own traumatic childhood experience and since his 30 or so years in clinical work with traumatised men, women and children he has been involved with the evolving science of the body/brain/relational field. Bessel Van Der Kolk uses a wide variety of therapeutic interventions in his Trauma Centres from Neurofeedback to retrain brain waves, to Yoga, Tai Chi and the arts including theatre, music, writing and painting. These are not all typical conventional treatments; however, they have all been researched and along with case studies show amazing results.

There is a movie, *Let There Be Light* made in 1946 that was commissioned to convince the public that shell shock veterans were healed and ready for a normal life, after having the treatment provided. It is a documentary directed by John Huston who was serving in the US Army Signal Corps during World War 11. The movie begins with war veterans returning back to US, where they enter a rehabilitation centre before returning to their hometowns.

Upon arrival these men are filmed with symptoms ranging from not being able to use their limbs to not being able to speak. They are an example of the impact of trauma. These men were young and healthy when they began their duty, and they all experienced similar traumas. It is clear that their reactions varied considerably. In the film, psychiatrists use a wide selection of therapies, from hypnotherapy, to group music and drama. The compassion and the insight of the psychiatrists makes the film seem like a magical journey from suffering to joy.

Bessel Van De Kolk, talks about this film in his book The Body Keeps The Score[5]. The movie reveals the connections made between their trauma symptoms and their childhood, it underlines the body mind connection and how trauma sees no boundaries in impact. After six months most of the men are ready to return to their lives and work. The narrator mentions how "Twenty percent of our army casualty suffered from post-traumatic symptoms, suffering from psychoneurotic symptoms, a sense of impending disaster, hopelessness, fear and isolation."[6]

The movie was suppressed from screening until the 1980's due to the 'unscripted presentation of mental disability'[7]. The government of the day saw this would impact on post war recruitment. Eventually with lobbying, the film was publicly released nearly 40 years later. One of the very clear indications of the movie was, the shattered self, could be reunited. Not from just one therapy, but with a variety of interventions done with kindness and compassion.

I was working on my body, my mind and my relationships with my room mates. It seemed odd but I did not want to talk to friends on the phone. I was at this point very sensitive to the vibrations that would keep me on an upward spiral and the outside world were not tuned into this experience of healing, that those around me were. Conserving my energy was key to limiting unnecessary stress. I wanted no distractions from the here and now, I needed the little energy I had to be connected to nurturing my healing self.

.

CHAPTER 5

The next two days were spent immersed in self-care. Breathing, prayer, affirmation, visualisations, tai chi/qigong and laughter, as well as avoiding stress. I was able at this point to put a pillow under my bottom and lift my knees up which would release pressure that was around my hips and back. I now had passed a bowel motion, in the bowl in bed. That was very embarrassing and close to humiliating. I was hoping I would not need to do this again, and so cut back on what I was eating, choosing either the soup or the meal at lunch but not both.

I could feel the difference day by day. Bettys snoring improved or I became used to it, and I no longer needed the 'endone' at night. The Pain Doctor came to see me. I told her what I was doing, and she was very impressed. She knew about the relationship between

Circadian Rhythms and healing, and told me she tells her patients to set their days with the sun and sleep with the dark, she said she was taking me off the 'endones,' that she could see from my face that I no longer needed them, and she was replacing them with anti-inflammatory and Paracetamol. When I asked her what she noticed just by looking at me, she said that usually the look on people's faces with my injury at this stage is white, no colour and full of tension, almost stone-faced, whereas I had colour in my face and was obviously relaxed.

This was interesting. I had become comfortable with the medication and fear was still very present, but the way this doctor spoke to me, tuning into my wavelength, I trusted her and was able to shift my fear of anticipatory pain without the endone, to relief.

I was improving, I could see round the corner. No longer did I need the medication for nausea, the anti-acid, the opioids. If I didn't relieve my bowels each day, they still gave me those tablets, sachets and the unpleasant liquid, however, I was getting closer to recovering.

I attempted to lift my head to see how far I could raise myself. Not much. I still could not have the electronic bed lift up more than slightly, I was still eating lying down on a slight slant. What I could see was that all the attentional breathing, tai chi, positional shifts, visualisations, affirmations, prayer and love (which I was feeling for my new brother and sister and what I called 'mothers', the nurses caring for us) was working, little by little. I noticed each slight extension and movement, the changes, and felt enormous gratitude to my body, my teachers, our creator and the enjoyable food.

I wanted to say thanks, so looked up the caterer who was in Melbourne and with a phone call was able to send my appreciation to the cook. Being kosher vegetarian and gluten free limited my menu options, but the food I did eat was delicious.

I waited for the neurosurgeon who came in the morning, the Indian gentle soul, who had supported my way of self-care as the dominant protocol, I wanted to thank him.

I had reached a new level of being, a sense of achievement ran through my system and I was further encouraged to move into the next stage. I increased the visualisations, to sitting up in the bed. I watched people in my sight, carefully, as they walked with ease, telling myself as I saw each person come and go, that soon, that will be me. I will sit up; I will walk again. All with ease, not with pain or the need for medication.

Eventually the 2 days passed and Thursday morning came. The birds came to the bare leafed tree every morning and afternoon. I enjoyed the waiting, the watching and the well-being that the birds displayed, the calm grace of the birds, swaying on the branch with the wind guiding its way. This was the day I needed to sit without the spasms and it had to be before the physio came.

After my routine, I used my hands to slowly walk step by step to support myself. With the slowness of my hands pressing into the bed pacing my lift, I could bring myself up, to a sitting position. No spasm, although at the sitting place there was an ache, a big ache. I counted to 5, then inching my hands down on the bed, back to the lying position I went. Bravo, I did it. I had sat up; I reached the goal. Breathing slow out breaths, I tried again. Now I was going to aim for 10 seconds. No, 5 was the limit.

I couldn't wait for both the neurosurgeon and the physio. The neurosurgeon was delighted, and said it must be my will power, he had never seen such recovery. The physio came, a different lady, and she said, 'swivel on the bed so your feet touch the floor'. That was a surprise, I hadn't even thought of setting a new goal. I was still impressed the spasms had stopped and I was counting my seconds sitting up. I was able to count to 10 before the achy pain started. Very slowly, I swiveled and very tentatively touched the ground, and no pain, then again, cautiously placed my feet without pressure just positioning them on the floor. "Look," she said, "your grounded."

Being grounded is a term meaning 'energetically

connected to the earth'. There is a perspective that sees our body as an 'electronic circuit' that represents a primary antioxidant defense system. Our bodies need to be in balance for our immune system to function and one of the key areas for balance is between the free radicals and antioxidants. Without this balance, chronic inflammation can result. Injuries, and the body's reactive system for repair, increase free radicals and hence the imbalance can occur. Temporary imbalance is necessary for fighting off damaged cells. Actually, the body is designed to restore imbalance. The problem is when the imbalance becomes chronic and the restoration doesn't occur. This was part of the research that Hans Selye worked on regarding the stress response.

Grounding, or walking with direct contact on the earth, is one of the ways that the body creates antioxidants activating all through the body. Just as plugging in an electric cord and switching it 'on', sends the electricity from the socket through the cord to the device. The body acts as the conduit when feet are on the ground, sending antioxidant activation though the body. When there is what Hans Selye called 'silent or smouldering' inflammation, the lack of antioxidants can create an inflammatory barricade, a wall of connective tissue surrounding a site of injury which can create an incomplete repair of the inflammation area and eventually the toxins can eventually cause impairment to the area or the system. Grounding, the direct contact with the earth is seen as being a way that antioxidants that come from the earth breakthrough the barrier that whole foods and exercise have not been able to.[1] This research indicates that grounding or earthing significantly alters the human bodies inflammatory response.

> "Selye studied the histology of the wall of the inflammatory pouch or barricade. It is composed of fibrin and connective tissue. Our hypothesis is that electrons can be semi-conducted across the barrier, and can then neutralize reactive oxygen species (free radicals). A semiconducting collagen pathway or corridor may explain how electrons from the Earth quickly attenuate chronic inflammation not resolved by dietary antioxidants or by standard medical care, including physical therapy. The barricade probably restricts diffusion of circulating antioxidants into the repair."[2]

> " Grounding appears to improve sleep, normalize the day–night cortisol rhythm, reduce pain, reduce stress, shift the autonomic nervous system from sympathetic toward parasympathetic activation, increase heart rate variability, speed wound healing, and reduce blood viscosity."[3]

One of the natural health modalities I work with is 'Shinrin Yoku' Nature Forest Therapy. This is now known as ecotherapy, forest therapy, nature therapy, forest bathing, grounding and earthing. I did an intensive course as a Nature Forest Therapy Guide,[4] and have practiced this modality working with children, adults as well as publishing articles on its health benefits and application.[5] Although going for a walk-in nature is not a modern idea, like many natural therapies, the benefits and practice of this self-care practice had been long forgotten. Rachel and Stephen Kaplan were Psychologists interested in nature benefits in the 1970s and eventually by 1989 their book, The experience of nature: A psychological perspective, offered the Attention Restoration Theory, (ART)[6] for understanding the psychological benefits of being and seeing nature.

With constant attention in processing information, the mind and body become fatigued, and ART, offers a way of restoring ourselves to a healthy rejuvenation. Research validates that nature offers the conditions for restoring our nervous system and these conditions, Rachel and Stephen Kaplan suggest include 'soft fascination'.

The difference between hard and soft fascination lies in the stimuli and to what extent we are actively brought into that stimulation. For example, hard fascination demands our full attention, we need to put effort into connecting to this stimulus, enough that our attention is focused. This is what can cause fatigue.

Think of the last time you watched a movie. No physical exertion but by the end of the movie, you yawn or ready for a nap. Conversely soft fascination is stimuli that takes our attention without entraining direct focus, little to no effort. This is what happens when you hear birds, or see a butterfly, watch the wind move through the leaves and branches. This soft attention leaves space for wondering, pondering and reflection, whilst hard fascination such as technology offers, is completely entraining. The pleasure of attending is critical to the restoration, and the colours, beauty and diversity of landscape naturally take us there.

I knew that looking out the window and seeing the clouds, sky, trees and birds, allowed my being to move into this place of healing. From my bed I could watch the colours of the sun set, and feel the soothing sense of calm flow through my body, doing good.

Yet, it took the Japanese to spark the research off to the physical benefits of walking in nature.

I was living in Japan in the early 1980s and was very much aware of how nature was integrated into urban life. The tatami mats, the floor coverings, were made of multi layered rice straw. Nobody wore shoes inside a home, or even in some restaurants. I remember accompanying a house mate to hospital by ambulance and fascinated at the importance of removing shoes. When the ambulance people arrived at our house, they quickly removed their shoes before entering our home, and we were all westerners living in this house, then, when they carried Anne out of the house, they stopped quickly to retrieve their shoes. Again, at the hospital, we all removed shoes before entering, there were lots of plastic slippers available but certainly it was protocol to never enter a place of residence or respect, with shoes on.

At this time, in the early 1980s' all the houses and apartments had tatami floor coverings. It was a few years later that carpet became popular. Under the foot, the soft earthly feeling of walking on nature was part of the different feeling that Japanese homes offered to foreigners. The temples that were abundant in Tokyo and other cities, incorporated nature as part of their distinctive features. I was more aware of the role nature has in city life in Japan than ever before, nature was inside, as well as outside. So, when I heard about 'Shirin Yoku' in 2016, I had a strong grasp on the context of why it would be taken seriously as a health initiative in Japan.

Shinrin Yoku began in Japan in the early 1980's as a government/ medical/ forestry response to *karoshi* which means death due to overwork. The research on karoshi is now accepted as part of modern society. This is currently a worldwide topic as the World Health Organisation, (WHO), working with International Labour Organisation (ILO) in their on-line news report, published May 2021, an article titled Long working hours increasing deaths from heart disease and stroke: WHO, ILO. identify:

> "The COVID-19 pandemic has significantly changed the way many people work, "said Dr Tedros Adhanom Ghebreyesus, WHO Director-General.

"Teleworking has become the norm in many industries, often blurring the boundaries between home and work. In addition, many businesses have been forced to scale back or shut down operations to save money, and people who are still on the payroll end up working longer hours. No job is worth the risk of stroke or heart disease. Governments, employers and workers need to work together to agree on limits to protect the health of workers....

"...Working 55 hours or more per week is a serious health hazard," added Dr Maria Neira, Director, Department of Environment, Climate Change and Health, at the World Health Organization. "It's time that we all, governments, employers, and employees wake up to the fact that long working hours can lead to premature death".[7]

The Japanese Government responded to karoshi, the work burnout/death syndrome awareness in 1983, by incorporating a 'forest bathing' culture, with guides and forest pathways into modern culture. Bringing together the Department of Forestry, and the health benefits of nature, the research into Shinrin Yoku began.[8] Almost twenty years later, a new department of ministry brought together Health, Labour and Welfare, in 2001 which makes decision making between work, health and welfare part of the same paradigm.

Self-Care the real story of healing

Dr Qing Li Physician and Immunologist at Nippon Medical School hospital in Tokyo, came to Japan in 1988 to study Japanese Advanced Medicine. Since that time, Qing Li has been studying and now teaching the effects of environmental chemicals, stress, and lifestyle on the immune function. He is currently the world's foremost expert in Forest Medicine and immunology. He established the new medical science known as Forest Medicine in 2012. Presently he is a physician at the Department of Rehabilitation and Physical Medicine, Graduate School of Medicine, Nippon Medical School, Tokyo, Japan.

Research now shows that forest bathing, impacts on our physical body by; improving cardiovascular function, hemodynamic indexes (heart and circulation), neuroendocrine indexes (tumour growth), metabolic indexes (overall body fitness/state), immunity and inflammatory indexes, antioxidant indexes, and electrophysiological indexes; significantly enhancing people's emotional state, attitude, and feelings towards things, physical and psychological recovery, and adaptive behaviours; and obvious alleviation of anxiety and depression.[9]

Putting my feet down on the 7th floor linoleum was not going to give me the medical benefit of earthing, or forest medicine, but it did remind me of how I was on the way to restoring my body towards well-being. I would again, sit under a tree and watch clouds go by, one of the many joys that I used to share with my grandchildren.

I thought that was enough for one day, to sit up and be 'grounded'. I spent the rest of the day practicing my sitting, working at extending the time, though I got to 10 and not beyond, as well as the other self-care practices. I was so happy; I could barely believe I had turned a corner. My room mates noticed the improvement, and we were all pleased. That night I tuned into more laughter, I had to do repeats but what was funny before still made me laugh.

The following morning a male physio came to see me, the doctor must have sought him out, as he introduced himself to me sharing his sukkot experience. It turned out I knew his parents, he and his brother attended the same school as my daughter at the same time, though different classes. Quickly trust was built between us, the connection was tangible as he invited me to walk with him. Walk, I was going to walk. The invitation was scary and exciting.

Carefully I sat up and rotated my legs to position them on the ground. He took my arm and even put his hand around my waist to give me the option of putting my weight on him if there was any problem. Carefully, slowly, with gentle deliberate deep breaths out, I touched the ground with my feet, lifting myself up from the bed allowing my weight to go to my feet. No pain, no tension, no ache, just strangeness.

For over a week I had not walked. It felt very new, even to the point of not being able to unconsciously just go. Instead, I reverted to a conscious thinking of what to do. I stood at first aware of no pain and then we decided to just have my hand above Bens[10] hand so if at any time of vulnerability, I could drop down to him for support. So off we went 'Follow the red line', Ben announced.

Heel, outside of foot. toe, right along the red line, then other foot, heal, outside of foot, toe, going down the red line. *"Is this how you usually walk?"* Ben asked, *"Well, I suppose not"*.. I realised that I was being very conscious in following directions. Walking on the red line and remembering the way I guide others to walk during a re-educating walking session with clients. I was actually needing to reeducate my feet to walk. The balance was scary, but Bens' presence created the safeness I needed to let go of the fear and walk, one foot in front of the other at a hips distance.

We were almost at the bathroom, a place I was eager to go by myself. *"Can I go here now? Do you think I can sit on the seat? I'm afraid."* We stopped at the bathroom, and with much apprehension I opened the door, and by myself entered. The commode was higher than the actual toilet so I positioned it and to my great surprise, no pain, a strange sense of being able to sit and release myself. Wow, I did it. Now, with more pride than fear I moved to the sink to wash my hands. Another wonderful experience, washing my hands. I re-joined Ben, and off we went slowly and carefully down the hall. I hadn't been here before, I could see the nurse's station, and the other ward rooms, and the busy ness of what was happening outside of what had been for the last week, my only vision. We walked to the end of the red line then back to my bed. It was such an exciting feeling, I continued on to have my first shower. Triumph, how great was that. I remembered hearing Betty say how wonderful it felt when she returned from the shower. Now it was my turn. It really was happening; the recovery was well on its way.

The hot water and the soap were refreshing. I realised I found it hard to move my hands the full extension and bending. One of my noticing's along this journey was how the muscles in my arms had wasted away to only flesh, no substance. When I began to do the Tai Chi in bed, I could see that my arms had lost all muscle tone, When I lifted my arms up there was no form just wasted skin, but after a few days of regular tai chi, the tone returned.

The regular day to day movements of washing myself had to be conscious so that my muscle actions could be edged towards reactivating my muscle memory.

I was exhausted. I returned to the bed. The nurse had put red socks on my feet before the physio therapists had come so now, I had wet socks. Bending down was not yet part of my capacity. With help from the nurse, to change into dry socks I was back on the bed recovering from a very strenuous morning. Robert and Betty applauded me. The journey truly had turned towards normality. It was now in sight.

The doctor arrived a bit later, this time it was not the Indian neurosurgeon. *"Hello, do you remember me? I was the neurosurgeon who first saw you down stairs, I'm sorry I haven't been here this week, I was on a conference."* He said. *"I hear your doing very well, you will go home on Monday."*

It hit me, had this neurosurgeon continued to be my doctor, I may not have had the recovery I had. He had made it clear that I was to be sent home with painkillers! I waited until he left, then with the realisation of the miracle of 'by chance', I started to cry. My tears flowed with deep release. I hadn't expressed the severity of my situation, I had from the beginning put my attention on positivity and healing thoughts, Now I realised how precarious my healing opportunity was. I was sure that I could not have made the decisions, the attention, the capacity of focus, if I had been at home. The distractions, the fear, the complexity of food, clothing, bedding, toileting, people taking my thoughts, energy in a very different direction.

I realised that the hospital is really a 'hospitable' environment as all these requirements for cleanliness and freshness are critical for well-being. At home these would all have been major details to be thought through and who would do them? There is no way I would have had clean sheets every few days, I don't even own that many sheets. I wash and put the same sheets on the bed. And as for toileting? How would that work??

Knowing treatment for diseases is not the only function of hospitals. The success of the functioning of the hospital comes from the environment as Florence Nightingale showed in the Crimean war of 1853. Her ideas revolutionised the hospital and nursing system valuing sanitation, cleanliness and kindness. Three things that sick people at home find very difficult to administer.

I was reminded of my next-door neighbour, Frank, who, after falling from his roof ended up in hospital with an operation to restore his collar bone. When he returned from his operation, he was on strong pain killers. His operation left him with an imbalance in his shoulders and little by little between the pain and his body change he became depressed. This led to more drugs and eventually he became drug addicted with not enough prescription satisfaction. He moved from a business man with a family of young children to being heavily in debt and estranged from his family. His commitment and attention were fully taken up by drugs, mostly illegal ones. Eventually he lost his home, his family and his business, finding himself homeless. I was familiar with the scenario as we were neighbours and many times I was involved in, 'emergencies.'

It occurred to me that I could easily have fallen through the cracks of a safety net into an addiction. The environment of the hospital, being away from home and taken care of, was part of my recovery. The ambiance of the hospital allowed me the space and time to focus on self-care in a way that the hustle and bustle of cooking, shopping, drop-in-friends, and busy life would not have supported. Instinctively I knew this.

The word hospital, comes from medieval Latin 'hospitale' – a place where guests are received. The earliest general hospital was built in 805 AD in Baghdad by Harun Al-Rashid, a political and religious leader. In indigenous and traditional societies around the world healing was an integral part of community living. For a society to survive someone had to have and pass on knowledge of therapeutic intervention, from childbirth to sickness to accidents, and this included mental health as well as physical, in fact for many indigenous societies there was no separation. Being happy and healthy went together.

Since human society began there have been healing traditions, learning what natural herbs heal what ailments, as well as traditional modalities such as cupping, which is known to be the oldest modality for healing.

Cupping was universal, using shells, leeches, as well as glass and today silicon.[11] By creating a suction, blood is forced into the area, increasing oxygen, hormones and infection fighters to flow, thus allowing impurities and toxins to be extracted through the circulation system. I remember when I studied cupping as a therapy, many years ago, I spoke to an elderly friend who was a holocaust survivor. I remember telling her about what I was studying and she told me, "oh yes, that was very common in Poland before the war. My father was a type of medic, not a doctor but in those days a doctor was not so common and very expensive. I would sometimes go with him when he was called out to do a 'banki'[12] treatment."

My training actually originated from an acupuncturist who came upon cupping in China, as this is probably one of the few places that still use cupping as a regular treatment for ailments by locals.

It is common to see modern health care being described as a Holistic theory. This is not a modern concept; it is actually the way indigenous society operated prior to colonialization and the introduction to reductionist thinking.

Richard Katz and Stephen Murphy-Shigematsu use the word synergy to describe the sense of all-inclusive, resulting in more than the sum of its parts.

> "Synergy refers to a pattern by which phenomena relate to one another, they come together, creating a new, greater and often unexpected whole from disparate, even conflicting parts. When synergy exists, resources become expanding, renewable, and widely accessible." [13]

Self-Care the real story of healing

Just as a short person needs to stand on the shoulders of another to reach up to oranges high on a tree, so synergy works via cooperation from different parts, resulting in two people together accessing the otherwise out of reach orange. The synergy of the hospital environment plus my self-care practices enabled my recovery. Either alone may not have produced the end result. The research on stress is clear that the body heals when the stress is alleviated.

The neurosurgeon told me that I would be going home on the Monday, in a few days' time. My tears shed for both the gratitude of serendipity that his conference inhibited him from sending me home with pain killers two days after my admittance to the hospital with a broken back, as well as gratitude that I had managed to get to the point of walking, showering, and at least momentarily sitting.

CHAPTER 6

My status as 'bed ridden', needing two nurses to move me, now changed. The chart next to the bed was rewritten and 'independent' was written across all criteria. I now was on a mission to walk, and began thinking of what I needed to do to live in my house.

I had to walk up and down steps, lift myself into and out of the bath, the shower was in the bath and my night-time ritual involves a soothing bath. I had to be able to dress myself, which included putting on my underpants and I needed to sit at different levels, including the toilet seat. My bathroom was too small to have any extra bits and pieces.

I asked a nurse if there were steps anywhere. I was shown the other end of the hall way where physio equipment was placed, chairs, stairs at various heights and railings. I had a new routine. I carefully walked up and down the hall 3 times, then over to the stairs, counting twenty times up and down. Initially holding onto the railings, and then after some time stepping without holding on. What was for so many years a mindless activity, walking, going up and down stairs, was now hard work. I was exhausted and needed to rest. Every hour I walked up and down. I could see each time, that it was a bit easier. I was that much more confident.

Betty was leaving for rehabilitation and Robert was going home to his wife. Although we were all a bit sad to say goodbye, each of us was grateful to continue our living experience, knowing how we had slowed down to a state we were happy to say goodbye to.

New people came and my new neighbour arrived with broken bones from her feet to her neck. She had been knocked over crossing a zebra crossing, and at her age of 80 years it had left her in a neck brace and a lot of pain. I was able to be of use now to the others in the room who were not able to move. I was recovering and could see my socialising stance shift more towards my usual way of looking at how I could be of service to others.

From a very young age I learnt that by helping people I helped myself. This past week in hospital had restrained me and I missed the feelings of connection that I had learnt come from caring for others. From experience I had found that waiting for someone to choose to connect to me could be a long wait, and very unpredictable, yet if I took opportunities to help or be of service to others, I increased my experiences of being connected. I spent a lifetime of practicing this art that needed balance so as not to move into unbalanced relationships or feelings of being taken advantage of.

Now I could raise myself out of bed, step out onto the floor, I could pass tissue boxes, move pillows, answer or pass phones. What appeared to be simple tasks were not simple for people who cannot reach out, or walk. Acts of kindness require more than emotional work; they also require able bodies. I looked for opportunities to practice getting out of bed. My movements were slow and careful, the fear of falling or of pain were still very present, and the more I practiced I could feel the power of my body returning.

I found the difference between flat in bed and upright offered very different perspectives of life. I wondered if babies have this sense of not being able to do much at all. I had talked about this at great length with Betty and Robert. We all felt the disempowerment that comes with immobility and yet our memories of having lived full mobile lives were very close to our identity.

Now that I was leaving the hospital yet still not fully

recovered, I was visited by an occupational therapist, a social worker and another physio therapist. They all wanted to support me in getting back to my previous lifestyle. It was decided that I would have 6 weeks of 'hospital at home', to start the day I get home. This would include 1 week of home rehabilitation and six weeks of three days a week a person to help with whatever I needed, for an hour each of the days.

My children insisted I should not be upstairs in my bedroom, and so I had my son take a mattress down to the 'treatment' room, where I usually practiced, for just a week. I had every intention of getting my life back to where it had left off, but I really had no idea if that was realistic. I still could not sit nor stand for long before aches would remind me of the need to lie down.

It was mixed feelings when the time came to leave. Mary, the lady next to me and I had shared many caring moments together. I was breathing with her, and although I could not stand next to her bed for an extended time, I did give her some energetic treatments to calm down her nervous system. I had from my own experience learnt the power of trauma, and its impact on the body. She even asked if I could stay longer, break another bone, in jest of course.

The day came, I was given medication, ten days of anti-inflammatory and paracetamol. although by now was taking no pills. One of the dear nurses took me downstairs with the beautiful pot of flowers that my sons' friend David had sent. These flowers had been a stunning surprise.

If you want to make someone smile, then give them flowers. That comes from research carried out by a group of academics whose conclusion found that 100% of the people who received flowers as opposed to food or other pleasing gifts, not only smiled sincerely but when followed up 3 days later still indicated a lift in mood.[1]

This their report said, is very unusual, to have 100% same reaction. They conclude it relates to evolutionary biology; humans being bred to enjoy flowers. I remember living in Hawaii, where everyone, ladies and men, wore garlands, leis around their necks and sometimes hair. This was mainly for celebrations, but locals often took a flower from a tree and put it behind their ear. It was one of the joys I discovered in life, that flowers made me smile.

After a few days in the hospital flowers for me had arrived and with them came a new identity. I was no longer just alone in a hospital bed; I was a loved person. The impact was immediate. The flowers were unusual, I don't know what they are called, nurses took photos so they could find others. The beautiful yellow mushroom like petals were just starting to open, and now 2 months later, they are still in bloom. I also received sun flowers, big and bright from my sister.

Hours after arriving home I was visited, neighbours

came to check what I needed, Sally Anne had organised food to come for the first two weeks, I had said I would manage, but when the food arrived daily, home cooked soups, fish, biscuits, rice, curry, challah (bread) it made eating so easy. The home visits began within hours with the physio therapist, Tom planning our appointments. I showed him the medication and asked if I should take it. His response was 'If you don't have pain, don't take pain killers which includes the anti-inflammatory, take them as needed, that is what they say."

In response to what can I do, "whatever doesn't hurt. If it hurts a bit, and you are still okay in a minute or so, then you're all good, if an ache or pain continues then stop."

Soon after the occupational therapist arrived. John was interested in my usual routine and supported me in sleeping upstairs.

I remember that as soon as I entered the gate of my house, I saw the flowers and overgrown weeds. As if they were welcoming me, I stood entranced at their presence. Opening the front door, the house looked so big. For nearly two weeks my home was a small table, that was all my 'things', now I was coming into a house with rooms, paintings, photos, memories of over half a century of collection.

I used to pride myself as a young person, that I owned so little. Travelling around the world for ten years, the only collection I had were memories. I didn't even have a camera. I would see material possessions as heavy, useless for someone who has to carry them. I remember when I began my parenting, home experience, the end of travelling and the beginning of a permanent residence, I moved with four boxes. Now, walking into my house in Bondi, it would take a removalist truck and I couldn't imagine how many boxes.

My son had done a good job in welcoming me home, he took out his ukulele and started playing. Home was a place where lots of things happen, people come and go, doors open and close and we can change the temperature by opening windows, putting on a fire or the gas heater or warming up soup. Empowerment was everywhere.

The nurse came while I was still in bed. I was now in the habit of spending most of the day in bed with short episodes of getting up to walk. The nurse took my blood, tested my oxygen level and blood pressure.

A few hours later John arrived, to take me on my first walk. Where would I like to go? I yearned to see the sea, and wild bush. Living in Bondi, my house was between Bondi Beach, Tamarama Beach and Bronte Beach. It was my habit until the injury to swim at Bronte Beach early mornings, or when the water got too cold, to walk the coastal path from Tamarama to Bondi.

"Let's go the flat footpath route to Mark's Park", the lookout that captures Bondi beach with sweeping ocean views. Neither of us were sure how long I would manage, and I was eager to find out. The physio wasn't able to come so it was the occupational therapist who was joining me. I felt a mix of apprehension, being cared for, and feeling invigorated with the outing. Slow walking is part of the conditions for nature therapy, and I had mastered the slow pace of movement since Rod Lee, who was the head of the Sydney Tibetan Society, had for the past few years been teaching me Tai Chi.

I was still consciously taking steps however, in the street, there were so many things to look at, my attention was diverted easily to flowers, to shrubs to the streetscape around us. We walked and walked and walked, we managed the full hour of his time with a slight dip in the road at one point.

To arrive at the sea was magical. Fresh air, the smell of the ocean the sounds of children playing in the park, birds singing and chirping. Then as if a show for us was created, a flock of birds above the water swept across the sky, then turned together in unison, to the other direction, and again, in unison as if dancing to a rhythm again to the opposite direction. They looked like shimmering sparkles of movement. I was back in my life, how amazing.

Today was an achievement. Full and tiring. My son warmed up our food. I was not very hungry, my appetite had not yet returned, however I could feel the love of homemade meals. Part of being in a religious community includes being part of wide circle of care. I had seen community working in many cultures in the world, mainly indigenous, that were based on shared beliefs. The core belief being caring for others. I had

Self-Care the real story of healing

witnessed people helping people in times of difficulty as well times of celebration. Just like the birds I had seen swooping across the Pacific Ocean at Bondi, I had witnessed how people coming together make the lives of others richer, sharing both pain as well as joy.

There were a few more tests I needed to try out with support. Getting into my own bath, and out again, walking on uneven ground, lying under a tree and getting up again. These were the movements that made my heart soft and gave me joy. The physio came and we tried these out and there was no pain, I just didn't feel the trust that I could do it alone.

Support came three times a week. It was not easy asking people to make my bed upstairs, do the ironing, wash the dishes, take the weeds out of the garden and clean the bathroom. I have never had a cleaner and to me these tasks were part of my self-care, I actually enjoyed the sense of caring for the areas I used. The level of care that I took was different from others. These people were not cleaners, they were 'hospital at home' support people. Again, I could see there were lots of things I needed to do that no one else would. I could see clearly the gap between how I was now and how I used to be and I was determined that the gap would diminish till I was where I wanted to be.

It was as if I was continuing on a journey of healing that revealed new goal posts. One of them was picking up my babies. Not my biological babies, but my grandchildren and a friend in the community's babies that I would look after when she needed the support. I had so much fear in creating pain, that I found it hard to go further. I could see I felt pain just picking up a glass of tea, so carrying anything was difficult, let alone a baby.

As days turned into weeks, I saw the changes. I found it hard to continue the level of self-care attention that I was able to focus on in the hospital. I couldn't with all the home distractions, it was impossible. I took to walking as much as I could, to lying on the floor with my feet on a chair to ease the ache when it came.

By four weeks I was back to swimming, first with side stroke, then with freestyle and eventually with breast stroke. There was no difficulty just the fear, 'Can I do this without causing injury?' I realised that although the water was not warm, I was able to have the courage to enter it and swim because I had years of experience in doing this. I remember clearly how I could enter the cold water knowing that in a short while I will be so immersed in the sea, the sense of connectedness that swimming offers, and that joy, the feeling of warmth on the inside will far outweigh the momentary splash of chill.

The earth is made up of approximately 70% water, just as we humans are made up of approximately 70% water. When we hear and see the ocean, a river or a waterfall we recognise a reflection of our own selves, an inner sense of well-being and nurturing as well as tears and thirst quenching. Some people identify themselves according the land, however there are many island people, and this includes indigenous people from all over the world, who link their genealogy via the sea, the water they come from. We cannot live without water; it is as important to our survival as much as food and air[2]. Our blood is made up of water, and this includes salt. The liquid that lubricates joints, sends out our hormones, digests our food, from our mouth to passing it out, as well as being the conduit for communicating to every cell in our body, regarding growth, nutrition and healing, includes water and salt. By swimming, or immersing and floating in the sea, the body is connecting with all our senses, including our inner mirror neurons that relate to the fractals.[3]

Fractals are the minute patterns of life that exist in all of nature, leaves, flowers, trees, even the clouds and water droplets. The fractals outside of us reflect the life that is inside of us. Our own mirror neurons connect with the safeness that comes with familiarity. We move into parasympathetic mode, that is a safe state, in nature, as long as this hasn't been interrupted by a trauma.

I didn't grow up swimming as a safe joyous state, but when I lived in Hawaii, it didn't take me long to tune into the soft warmth that the sea offered, and feel the gentle breeze soothe my soul. I learnt there, the value of the ocean, the healing sound, the warmth of soothing rhythm nurturing my body, mind and soul.

Hot springs, mineral baths, and hot water bathing was part of European culture with the Romans, Ottomans, Persians and Arabs taking these over the world as they colonised all parts of the globe. It was not only pleasurable but well known for healing. It was called thalassotherapy, 'thalass' meaning sea water.

> "Ocean water differs from river water in that it has significantly higher amounts of minerals, including sodium, chloride, sulphate, magnesium and calcium..,,, Cold-water swimming activates temperature receptors under the skin that release hormones such as endorphins, adrenalin and cortisol."[4]

As I regained my swimming, the courage of entering the water when the weather was still not warm, crept into other areas. I started carrying shopping, picking up the bag of wet washing to hang on the line. Bit by bit the relationship with my back changed from fear to courageous care. One day I bent down and pulled-out weeds in the garden and, no pain, no problem.

At six weeks from coming home, the hospital at home ended and although I am not completely as I was, I am back to mostly all. Even picking up the children. Not as before where I would put them on the baby carrier/sling and carry them for hours on my back or front, but long enough to calm the baby, long enough to soothe the sighs.

Self-care is still a priority for me, the early morning swims in the ocean, tai chi daily, and lying, in various positions that totally soothe any aches in my back.

Self-Care the real story of healing

They say prevention is better than cure, from my experience I would say prevention is preparation for cure.

ABOUT THE AUTHOR

Michelle Brenner was born in the late 1950's and although was raised in a Jewish home had a mother who was involved in yoga and meditation. Michelle grew up with a strong awareness of otherness. As a child in the 60's she was taken to a Naturopath when she were sick, attended yoga and meditation classes as an observer and even spent weekends at an ashram. Michelle travelled around the world from a teenager, being very interested in how other people lived especially those close to nature. She lived in Hawaii, Japan, Indonesia as well as New Zealand, France, Israel, England and Scotland.

She studied Natural Health Therapy and had a career in Conflict Resolution as a mediator, community facilitator and teaching Assertive Communication, Mediation, and Cross-Cultural Communication.

She now practices holistic health using body/mind modalities. She has 2 children and 2 grandchildren.

She has 2 other books on Amazon.com Conscious Connectivity Creating Dignity in Conversation and Conversations on Compassion. Both these books include contributions for a variety of authors. She has many published articles some of these can be found at https://www.mediate.com/author/Michelle-Brenner/1086
contact details; brennermichelle@hotmail.com

Michelle Brenner

ENDNOTES

Chapter 1

[1] Jon Kabat Zinn <u>Full Catastrophe Living: Using the Wisdom of Your Body and Mind to Face Stress, Pain, and Illness</u> published by Little Brown Book Group Carmelite House 2013

[2] Bridget Grenville-Cleave, Dóra Guðmundsdóttir, Felicia Huppert, Vanessa King, David Roffey Sue Roffey, Marten de Vries <u>Creating The World We Want To Live In How Positive Psychology Can Build a Brighter Future</u> Routledge Press 2011

Chapter 2

[11] Herbert Benson <u>The Relaxation Response</u> reprinted 2001 William Morrow publ. px

[2] Ibid Herbert Benson pxi

[3] Ibid Herbert Benson pxii

[4] Ibid Herbert Benson pxiiii

[5] Satchin Panda https://singjupost.com/health-lies-in-healthy-circadian-habits-satchin-panda-at-tedxbeaconstreet-transcript/

[6] Satchin Panda <u>The Circadian Code</u> pxvii Rodale publ 2018

[7] Emily NC Manoogian and Satchidananda Panda <u>Circadian rhythms, time-restricted feeding, and healthy aging</u> Ageing Res Rev. 2017 Oct; 39: 59–67. Published online 2016 Dec 23 https://www.ncbi.nlm.nih.gov/pmc/articles/PMC5814245/

[8] Satchin Panda <u>The Circadian Code</u> Rodale publ. 2018
[9] K.Straif et al, "<u>Carcinogenicity of Shift-Work, Painting, and Fire-Fighting</u>" Lancet Oncology 8 no12 (2007)
[10] Satchin Panda ibid 2018 p52
[11] Satchin Panda ibid 2018 p98,99
[12] Christine M. Swanson, M.D., Wendy M. Kohrt, Ph.D., Orfeu M. Buxton, Ph.D., Carol A. Everson, Kenneth P. Wright, Jr., Eric S. Orwoll, M.D., and Steven A. Shea, Ph.D. <u>The Importance of the Circadian System & Sleep for Bone Health</u> Published online 2017 Dec 9 10 1016/i.metabol.2017 12 002
[13] Chao Song, Jia Wang, Brett Kim, Chanyi Lu, Zheng Zhang, Huiyong Liu, Honglei Kang, Yunlong Sun, Hanfeng Guan, Zhong Fang, and Feng Li <u>Insights into the Role of Circadian Rhythms in Bone Metabolism: A Promising Intervention Target?</u> Published online 2018 Sep 27. Biomed Res Int. 2018; 2018: 9156478.

Chapter 3

[1] Daniel Siegel <u>Pocket Guide to Interpersonal Neurobiology</u> 2012 Norton and Company publ. chapters 11,19 and 23
[2] Editor: Alexander Muacevic and John R Adler Bruno Bordoni, Shahin Purgol, Annalisa Bizzarri, Maddalena Modica, and Bruno Morabito <u>The Influence of Breathing on the Central Nervous System Monitoring</u> Published online 2018 Jun 1. doi: 10.7759/cureus.2724
[3] James Nestor <u>Crooked teeth? Your ancestors chewed 4 hours every day</u>

https://www.youtube.com/watch?v=YO_UecN2DiM March 2021

[4] Cannon, Walter <u>Bodily Changes in Pain, Hunger, Fear and Rage: An Account of Recent Researches Into the Function of Emotional Excitement</u>. FQ Legacy Books 2010 p.326

[5] Dr Hans Seyle 2010 https://www.youtube.com/watch?v=WxcTEiTrS0k and <u>Hans Selye (1907–1982): Founder of the stress theory</u> Siang Yong Tan, MD and A Yip, Singapore Med J. 2018 Apr; 59(4): 170–171.

[6] Dr Hans Seyle 2010 https://www.youtube.com/watch?v=WxcTEiTrS0k

[7] Herbert Benson Ibid 2001 xvii

[8] Sydney University News. Nov 2019 https://www.sydney.edu.au/news-opinion/news/2019/11/20/you-know-medicines-placebo-effect-now-meet-the-nocebo-effect.html

[9] https://blog.apsoc.org.au/2019/10/04/understanding-placebo-and-nocebo-effects-a-chat-with-ben-colagiuri/comment-page-1/

[10] https://drdavidhamilton.com/the-science-of-high-performance-in-sport/

[11] Neeta Mehta Mind-body Dualism: <u>A critique from a Health Perspective</u>   March 2011 https://www.researchgate.net/publication/51240134_Mind-body_Dualism_A_critique_from_a_Health_Perspective

[12] Neeta Mehta Ibid

[13] Neeta Mehta Ibid

[14] https://positivepsychology.com/broaden-build-theory/

[15] Barbara Fredrickson Love 2.0 Finding Happiness and Health in Moments of Connection pub Plume 2013
[16] David Hamilton How Your Mind Can Heal Your Body publ Hay house 2018 p 87
[17] Timothy Speicher Positional Release Therapy Institute and David Draper Brigham Young University - Provo Main Cam Top-10 Positional-Release Therapy Techniques to Break the Chain of Pain, Part 1 September 2006 Athletic Therapy Today
[18] Colin Ross MD. Human Energy Fields: A New Science and Medicine 2009 Manitou Communications
[19] Ming Zhang, Mohamed Moalin, Lily Vervoort, Zheng Wen Li, Wen Bo Wu, and Guido Haenen Connecting Western and Eastern Medicine from an Energy Perspective Published online 2019 Mar 26.. https://www.ncbi.nlm.nih.gov/pmc/articles/PMC6470590/
[20] Roger Jahnke, OMD, Linda Larkey, PhD, Carol Rogers, Jennifer Etnier, PhD, and Fang Lin A Comprehensive Review of Health Benefits of Qigong and Tai Chi First Published July 1, 2010 Review Article Find in PubMed https://doi.org/10.4278/ajhp.081013-LIT-248 and https://undsci.berkeley.edu/article/acupuncture
[21] R. I. M. Dunbar, Rebecca Baron, Anna Frangou, Eiluned Pearce, Edwin J. C. van Leeuwen, Julie Stow, Giselle Partridge, Ian MacDonald, Vincent Barra, and Mark van Vugt Social laughter is correlated with an elevated pain threshold Proc Biol Sci. 2012 Mar 22; 279(1731): 1161–1167. Published online 2011 Sep 14.
[22] Three Emotion Regulation Systems Compassion Focused Therapy THREAT, DRIVE, SOOTHING

#LewisPsychology
https://www.youtube.com/watch?v=L-GQPOJWOrI.
[23] Dr Paul Gilbert Compassion: <u>From Its Evolution to a Psychotherapy</u> December 2020 Frontiers in Psychology 11
[24] Deb Dana <u>The Polyvagal Theory in Therapy Engaging the Rhythm of Regulation</u> Published by Norton Professional Books 2020
[25] Stephen W. Porges PhD The <u>polyvagal theory: New insights into adaptive reactions of the autonomic nervous system</u> Cleveland Clinic Journal of Medicine February 2009, 76 (4 suppl 2) S86-S90;

Chapter 4

[1] <u>Japanese Zen Buddhist Philosophy</u> First published Wed Jun 28, 2006; substantive revision Wed Jul 31, 2019
https://plato.stanford.edu/entries/japanese-zen/
[2] https://en.wikipedia.org/wiki/%C3%89mile_Cou%C3%A9 Marguerite Marshall. "<u>Applied Auto-Suggestion of Famous French Healer Explained.</u>" Boston Post, January 4, 1923, p. 13 and quoted by Frederick L. Collins, "Three Minutes With a Headliner." (Kingston Jamaica) The Gleaner, February 9, 1923, p.6.
[3] Gabor Mate
https://www.youtube.com/watch?v=nmJOuTAk09g
[4] Bessel Van Der Kolk <u>The Body Keeps The Score</u> Penguin 2014
[5] Ibid Bessel Van Der Kolk 2014

[6] Let There Be Light
https://www.filmpreservation.org/preserved-films/screening-room/let-there-be-light-1946
[7] Let There Be Light Wikipaedia

Chapter 5

[1] Georgia Kinch <u>Body-Earthing</u> publ. The Psychology of Extraordinary Beliefs Ordinary students exploring extraordinary beliefs Ohio State University 2018
https://u.osu.edu/vanzandt/2018/04/18/body-earthing/
James L Oschman, Gaétan Chevalier, and Richard Brown <u>The effects of grounding (earthing) on inflammation, the immune response, wound healing, and prevention and treatment of chronic inflammatory and autoimmune diseases</u> J Inflamm Res. 2015; 8: 83–96. Published online 2015 Mar 24.
https://www.ncbi.nlm.nih.gov/pmc/articles/PMC4378297/
https://www.researchgate.net/figure/Formation-of-the-inflammatory-barricade-Notes-Copyright-C-1984-Selye-H-Reproduced_fig4_274644091
Davis Langdon <u>Bioelectromagnetic and Subtle Energy Medicine</u> Routledge; 2 edition 2014

[2] James Oschman, Gaetan Chevalier, Richard Brown Ibid
https://www.ncbi.nlm.nih.gov/pmc/articles/PMC4378297/

[3] James Oschman et al Ibid

[4] Association of Nature Forest Therapy Guides and Programs
https://www.natureandforesttherapy.earth/

[5] https://www.mediate.com/author/Michelle-Brenner/1086,

https://www.resurgence.org/magazine/author1988-michelle-brenner.html,

[6] Stephen Kaplan The restorative benefits of nature: Toward an integrative framework 1995 Science Direct https://www.sciencedirect.com/science/article/abs/pii/0272494495900012

[7] https://www.who.int/news/item/17-05-2021-long-working-hours-increasing-deaths-from-heart-disease-and-stroke-who-ilo

[8] Qing Li Editor Forest Medicine - Public Health in the 21st Century Nova Science Publ. 2013

[9] Ye Wen, Qi Yan, Yanglui Pan, Xinren Gu, Yuangqui Liu Medical empirical research on forest bathing (Shinrin-yoku): a systematic review Environmental Health and Preventive Medicine Dec 2019 https://environhealthprevmed.biomedcentral.com/articles/10.1186/s12199-019-0822-8

[10] I am not sure if he is called Ben, but I do remember his last name as Cantori

[11] https://www.physio-pedia.com/Cupping Therapy

[12] Polish word for cupping.

[13] Richard Katz PhD, Stephen Murphy-Shigematsu PhD Synergy, Healing, and Empowerment: Insights from Cultural Diversity Brush Education Inc. publ 2012

Chapter 6

[1] Jeannette Haviland-Jones, Holly Hale Rosario, Patricia Wilson, Terry R. McGuire An Environmental Approach to Positive Emotion: Flowers Evolutionary Psychology, vol. 3, 1, First Published Jan 1, 2005

[2] https://www.usgs.gov/special-topic/water-science-school/science/water-you-water-and-human-

body?qt-science_center_objects=0#qt-science_center_objects
[3] https://womenandwavessociety.com/8-reasons-why-being-in-on-or-around-water-makes-you-feel-so-good/
[4] https://theconversation.com/health-check-why-swimming-in-the-sea-is-good-for-you-68583

Manufactured by Amazon.com.au
Sydney, New South Wales, Australia